MIND YOUR BRAIN

How to help your brain stay healthy into old age

Brigitte de Lange

ACKNOWLEDGMENTS

With thanks to my husband Don, for his unconditional support and his interest, while listening to relentless accounts of the wonders of the brain

With thanks to our dog Wifey who showed endless patience when again there was no time to play ball and only let out an occasional heavy sigh

With thanks to all the healthy and content octogenarians and nonagenarians I have come to know, especially Willy, Wouter, Margaret, and Herman, who are living proof of the fact that it is possible to age gracefully and be happy into very old age

CONTENTS

PREFACE

I have always had a weak spot for older adults. It is so much easier to be young. You still have your whole future ahead and have a world of possibilities open to you to make choices and set out on your way.

Reaching the end of life, for many elderly it is hard to stay optimistic. The world in general seems to be far worse off than it was in their 'good old days'. Young people are far too occupied to care about their older fellow human beings. And for the old adults themselves only death lies ahead, probably preceded by disease and surely by a decline in capabilities.

I feel pity for the older persons around me and compassion. Many of them seem sad and depressed, not satisfied with life as it is now for them and reminiscing about what used to be or about chances they had missed and things they would have liked to do differently.

The resilient and adaptable me rebels against the idea that this is the only way it can be. I don't want to resign to the fact that it is the destiny of elderly to have their lives just fizzle out. Why can't this last phase of life be exciting and rewarding, making use of all the wisdom one has gathered and not having to worry anymore about careers and social status?

In many cases, health problems put a spoke in the wheel. Pensioners have the time to do all kinds of interesting things, but aches and pains, illnesses, and a lack of energy frequently keep them from doing so.

But then again, you see some older adults enjoying good health and a great range of physical, social, and mental abilities. What is making the difference and how do these people succeed in ageing well? Not everyone getting old will become infirm. And certainly not every older person will suffer dementia. Lifestyle, social, and psychological factors are linked with health in older adults.

I set out to investigate the effects of brain training. I started my research based on the hypothesis that mental training would be the ultimate tool to keep the brain healthy and stave off age-related diseases like dementia. It seemed like the egg of Columbus.

But the more my research advanced, the less unambiguous the information became. Yes, it is good to activate your brain, especially in elderly who sometimes just doze away literally and figuratively. Yes, the brain does show plasticity in adapting networks and connections with use. But is doing brain games on the computer really helping your brain to stay healthy and improve memory?

The answer is 'no', not just like that. I had to conclude mental training is an added value. It is important, but not indispensable. It may be third on the list after the right kind of nutrition. The only real thing is physical activity. Working out your body has a huge protective effect on your brain.

The message is clear: if we want to keep our cognitive abilities functioning well into old age, we have to start and keep on moving!

Now, I made it my life's goal to spread this message. It seems such a shame to let pass the opportunity of a brilliant old age just because we haven't taken care of our brain. Especially since the steps to take are that simple. But exercising is probably the least favourite activity of mankind nowadays. We invent all kinds of substitutes that won't work just to avoid getting ourselves in motion. But doesn't this strain seem trivial compared to the magnificent result of a well-functioning brain and as a matter of course a well-functioning body as well?

So, read this manual, start implementing the recommendations, and gradually make your lifestyle more brain-conscious. Your wonderful brain deserves it!

Brigitte de Lange

INTRODUCTION

OLDER AND BETTER

What could be more fascinating than our brain? It produces the most fantastic thoughts. Everything we know about worlds as far away as other solar systems or as small as an atom has once been discovered by an inquisitive brain. Even the knowledge we have about the brain itself has derived from the researching brains of driven scientists.

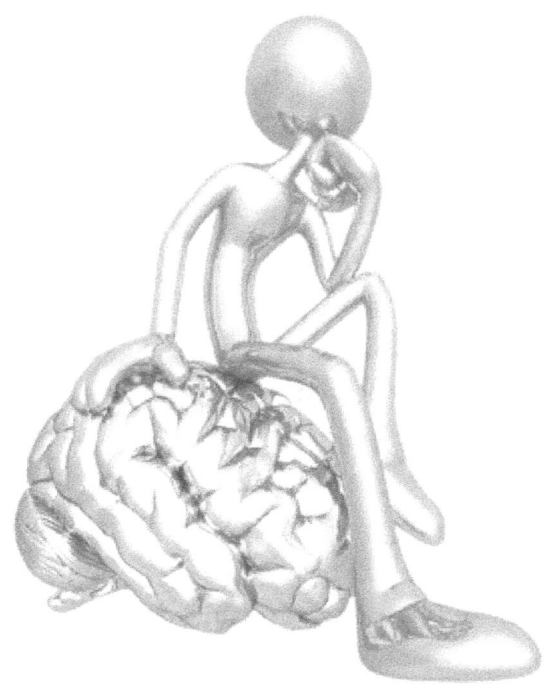

(© Scott Maxwell - Fotolia.com)

Everything we know about the brain has derived from the researching brains of driven scientists. So much has changed recently regarding our knowledge of this amazing organ. Findings assumed to be facts during the early years of brain research have turned out to be wrong. This is quite understandable since those early brain scientists had to work with very limited resources. Their lab equipment was nowhere near the state-of-the-art tools that are available nowadays. Although the microscope had been in use for a couple of hundred years, still it took until the end of the 19th century before scientists could see a brain cell, the neurone, through it for the first time. And they had to wait another hundred years before they could study live brain cells in action with the help of scanning equipment.

For many decades, scientists had no doubts about certain brain facts. The brain, supposedly, was laid down rather definitively at birth. We were born with all the neurones we were going to get. During our lifetime, neurones only died at a rapid pace and no new ones were born. The brain didn't have an inbuilt capacity to recover either.

In no more than two decades, all these certainties were thrown overboard. They have proven to be false and we have had to radically revise our ideas. More sophisticated research technologies shed a whole different light on the brain and all its powers. Our knowledge of the human brain has grown explosively. New findings do not fail to amaze us. And according to people in the know we have only scratched the surface. Many more developments and discoveries will follow.

Every new finding only adds to the list of questions we still have about the functioning of the brain. It becomes ever more clear how complicated our brain is. It is an intricate sum of many, many items and processes such as brain cells, chemicals and electric currents. What happens in one part of the brain influences what is going on in other parts. When you tinker with one section another section will suffer the consequences. There's a lot to be discovered before we will have a more complete picture of the workings of our brain, let alone build a complete brain from scratch.

Knowledge

We should be extremely grateful for the brain we ended up with through the evolution of mankind. Not only did nature make sure it is safely tucked away in our skull, but it is also capable of extraordinary achievements. Our brains can adapt to circumstances in an impressive way and they have an unlimited capacity to learn. From one generation to the next, we continue to know more. A child being born at this moment does not have to invent the wheel all over again, but can just use all the knowledge that has been gathered in past centuries.

The human brain is able to constantly come up with new ideas, also founded on knowledge acquired by brains in times long gone by. This is only possible thanks to the brain's capacity to share information with other brains; at first, through sounds and gestures, then via spoken language and afterwards in a far bigger and more lasting way through written language. In this way, through the course of time, a kind of gigantic 'universal brain' has come into being which every newcomer of the human race can tap into and also add new facts to.

The average person doesn't know a whole lot about how his

brain functions. A lot of information has been given about for instance ways to keep your heart healthy or what to do to strengthen your bones. The importance of keeping a healthy weight and products to lose weight are in the spotlight. But brain awareness is lacking behind. The brain, however, deserves far more interest since it is precisely our brain that governs the rest of our body.

Adaptability

The brain is an incredibly flexible organ that improves with use. The more you put your brain to work the better it functions. It becomes more efficient and opens up room for new tasks. In that way, our brain does not resemble a machine which will deteriorate through frequent use despite being well-oiled and maintained.

The brain is incredibly flexible, improves with use and has the capacity to share information with other brains.

The brain also has an amazing power to adapt to changing circumstances. It makes sure we can survive and function well in extremely different environments. But even when something goes wrong in our head, due to a stroke for instance, the brain is so adaptable it has the possibility to regroup brain cells to continue functioning as normal as possible.

Nevertheless, our brain is very vulnerable too. Precisely because it is such a complex entity, the delicate balance inside our skull can easily be disrupted. A minimal change could have devastating consequences for the well-being of large parts of the brain. A tiny problem could start a chain reaction and thus cause a dramatic decline in our cognitive abilities.

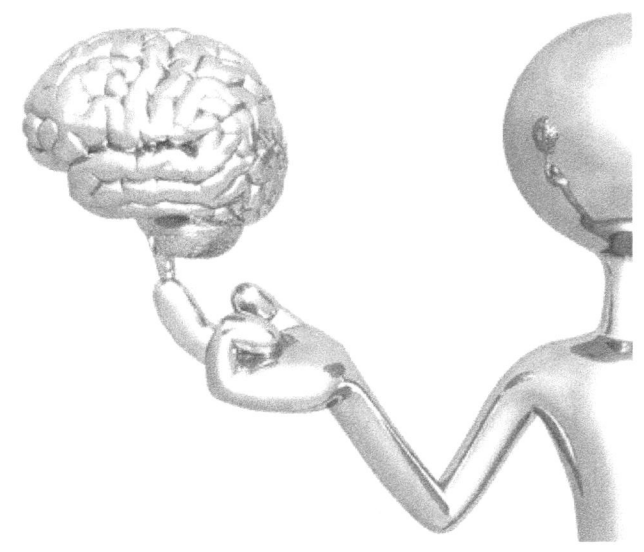

(© Scott Maxwell - Fotolia.com)

Fate

People are getting older, although unless science proves otherwise there is a limit to this growth in age. Maximum life span is the maximum number of years an organism can live. For human beings, maximum life span is about 120-125 years. Life expectancy is the number of years probably lived by the average person born in a particular year. For thousands of years, human life expectancy stayed at 32-45 years.

In the 20th century, life expectancy has increased considerably. It has risen up to around 80 years in many countries in the developed world. The number of centenarians worldwide is estimated close to 500,000, according to the United Nations. The majority of centenarians live in the United States and Japan. Some experts think the number of centenarians will reach nearly 6 million in 2050. This rise is mainly thanks to reduction in infant mortality, better nutrition, development of vaccines and antibiotics, and advances in treatment and prevention of heart disease and stroke.

But research shouldn't only be about lengthening life. Attention also has to be paid to maintaining and enhancing its quality. The older we get, the higher our chance of getting age-related diseases, such as cardiovascular disease, arthritis, osteoporosis, and type 2 diabetes. Also degenerative brain diseases like Alzheimer disease and Parkinson disease mainly occur in elderly people. These brain diseases typically go hand in hand with dementia, a cluster of disorders that result in cognitive decline.

Nowadays, when there's talk about ageing it's almost always about problems regarding the ageing population. It seems like dementia is hanging like the sword of Damocles over everybody's head who dares to reach an advanced age. But dementia certainly is not an inescapable destiny. The fact that more and more people are affected by dementia is firstly because more people reach the ages when the dementia risk is getting higher. But other factors also play a role since not only the absolute numbers of elderly suffering dementia are growing, but also the percentage of dementia sufferers per age group.

Scientific research comes up with ever more evidence that lifestyle is one of the main culprits in the rise of dementia. Apparently, it is the way we live that makes us more susceptible to a decline in cognitive functioning. So, it's high time to get to know a bit more about what is happening in our brain when we age, what dementia does to our brain and most importantly, what we can do to prevent dementia.

Lifestyle

In the past, people didn't have to think about how to keep their brains healthy since that happened automatically. They lived their lives at a more relaxed pace and in a more natural way. Besides, most people didn't become old enough to run the risk of dementia.

Even though we do reach far more advanced ages now, that doesn't mean we always have to get health problems and go downhill. We do hold all the trump cards in our hand to make our final life stage a pleasant and interesting one. After all, having reached old age, we don't have to worry anymore about our social position or our career and we have gathered a huge amount of experience and wisdom. But we have to make sure to adapt our lifestyle to help our brain stay in the best condition possible.

What follows in Mind Your Brain is a practical guide to take destiny into your own hands. What actions can you take to contribute to the health of your brain? What happens in the brain when we get older? Why might we be affected by dementia? What can we do ourselves to minimise the risk of dementia? The answers to these questions and the accompanying explanation are based on the latest state of affairs in brain research.

The good news is you can throw those dull computer games with which you should train your brain, out of the window. You don't have to be upset either about a few pounds of overweight. The bad news is you really do have to get out of that couch in front of the television or step away from your computer screen to keep your brain healthy. Exercise is the most important part of living brain-consciously.

PART I THE BRAIN

We don't spend many thoughts on that grey mass – which in reality isn't grey but a soft pink – in our head. Other parts of our body usually occupy our minds more often. Bellyache, backache, sore muscles, fatigue: signals from our body with which we are all too familiar. Of course we know it is the brain that governs the whole of our body, but that hardly ever enters our mind. We just assume that the brain does what it must do and above all does that correctly.

Most of the time that is indeed the case. The way our brain keeps on functioning and almost never lets us down in our busy daily life is amazing. Day in day out, the brain makes sure our body functions like a well-oiled machine. If something goes wrong somewhere, the brain directs the repair. It does its job so perfectly, we never think about whether all is well up there in that brainpan. A thought, by the way, that would also be produced by that same brain. Even when we don't take very good care of ourselves, our brain tries to keep the machine running as long as possible. It is incredible how much we can undermine our health without anything actually going very wrong.

Unfortunately, some attacks on our body cells do pile up. In the beginning, you don't notice anything, but yet more damage can't be casually smoothed away by the brain anymore. At advanced age, you may be presented with the bill for a reckless lifestyle during your young years for example. But even then, the brain is so potent and flexible that it can take emergency measures and improve quite a lot of the malfunctions. It is up to you to help the brain with this daunting task by adhering to a healthy, brain-conscious lifestyle.

To be able to live brain-consciously it is important to have at least some insight into the architecture of the brain and its workings.

1. TWO FISTS

What's inside our skull?

Our brain is about the size of two clenched fists and it weighs less than 3 lbs. (1.5 kilograms). The brain consists of two parts: a right half and a left half called cerebral hemispheres.
The brain consists of two intensely cooperating halves, the left and right cerebral hemispheres.

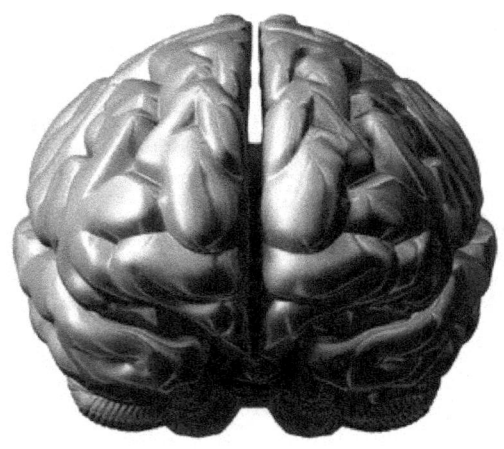

(© diez-artwork - Fotolia.com)

The left hemisphere in principle governs the right side of the body and the right hemisphere the left side. Someone who had a stroke in his left hemisphere could become paralysed in for instance his right arm or leg. Such a stroke is due to a disturbance in the blood flow to the brain. This can be the result of a blockage or a haemorrhage. A cerebrovascular accident hardly ever happens in both hemispheres at the same time. If a paralysis does affect both sides of the body, this is generally caused by damage to the spinal cord.

Even though the two hemispheres are responsible for different parts of the body they do work together intensely all the time. During evolution, hemispheric specialisation occurred because it was an advantage having two different forms of representations, but both hemispheres usually contain the essential machinery for performing all tasks. The hemispheres are connected via the corpus callosum. This is a kind of master cable in the centre of your head made up of nerve fibres coming from both hemispheres. The corpus callosum makes information exchange between the left and right hemispheres possible.

In some people, this connection between both hemispheres is broken. In exceptional circumstances for instance the cable is cut surgically. This is done sometimes if a person suffers an extreme form of epilepsy and all other possible treatments have failed. In most cases, the number of epileptic seizures decreases considerably after surgery. The patient ends up having a split-brain.

Split-brain is not only the term used for people having undergone the operation to sever the corpus callosum, but is also in fact the real consequence of the procedure.

Experiments involving persons with a split brain showed that both hemispheres have their own consciousness. Since the hemispheres are not connected and cannot consult one another, they both come up with their own explanation of an activity. That story is not unambiguous. The right hemisphere appears to stick to the facts to a greater extent, whereas the left hemisphere loses itself quickly in speculation to try to make a logical whole out of events. In people who have a normal functioning corpus callosum, there could exist the possibility, the sober right hemisphere keeps the unbridled interpretations of the left hemisphere in check to a certain degree.

This does not mean it would be useful to accept invitations for training programs to find out which of the two is your dominant hemisphere, to develop your right hemisphere more, or to bring both your hemispheres in balance. So far, no scientific evidence has come up to corroborate the improvements these programs promise.

Walnut

Both hemispheres are essentially the same. Both contain the elemental machinery to accomplish all the necessary tasks. During evolution, a certain specialisation took place, since it turned out to be useful to look at the world in different ways. One of those specialisations concerns language. In almost all human beings, the left hemisphere is dominant where language is concerned. This applies even to left-handed people in whom you would expect the opposite since the left side of the body is governed by the right hemisphere. In only a small percentage of left-handed people, the right hemisphere is dominant for language. One of the specialisations of the right hemisphere concerns spatial manipulation.

Both hemispheres are made up of the same parts. The upper layer consists of the cerebral cortex. Thanks to its typical twists, it makes the brain look like a giant walnut. It probably happened during evolution that the cortex started twisting.

This way, more of the cortex' neural tissue fits in the limited area of the skull. Only large mammals have a folded cortex. In smaller animals it has a smooth appearance.

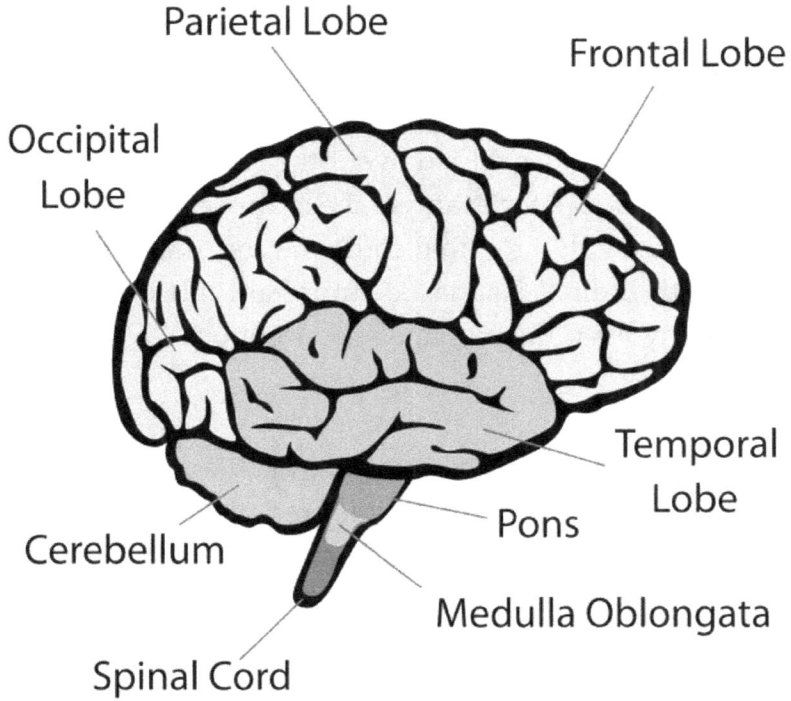

(© Athanasia Nomikou - Fotolia.com)

Important sections of the brain. Both brain halves consist of the same areas.

The cortex incorporates different areas for different tasks. One part for instance is responsible for movement, the motor cortex. Another part receives information from the senses, the sensory cortex. This is where images that enter via our eyes and sounds that enter via our ears are being processed. A very important part of the cortex is the prefrontal cortex, which is situated in the anterior part of the brain, right behind the forehead. In the prefrontal cortex, all those important actions take place that make us feel human. It presides over our thought processes and is responsible for such things as planning, decision making and our social behaviour.

The cerebral cortex lies folded over other important structures. These are for example the brainstem, which forms the connection with the spinal cord, and the cerebellum – Latin for little brain – that has an important role in movement, but is also involved in language and attention.

Seahorse

Of course it is possible to make a very detailed subdivision of both hemispheres. But the nice, coloured pictures from hemispheres with all the different parts you find on the internet haven't got a lot to do with reality. Looking at the pulp on the counter in the research laboratory you can hardly find any subdivision. Although the history of brain research is relatively short, beautiful maps of the brain have been made thanks to persistent researchers. These maps not only show the different parts of the brain, but in many cases also combine them with certain functions performed by those parts.

Already in the beginning of the 20th century, the German neurologist Korbinian Brodmann subdivided the cerebral cortex into 52 areas, which he all gave a name and a number. Nowadays, this numbering is still used. When reading about the brain, you frequently encounter references to Brodmann areas.

Over the years though, it turned out some parts of the brain don't really belong together as far as actual contacts and functional cooperation are concerned and other parts do. Modifications to the division of the brain we use are ongoing. An indisputable fact is that all the different parts of the brain, no matter which names we give them, together form a large, integrated whole.

I would like to put one small brain part in the spotlight here, since it plays such an essential role in the proper functioning of the brain at advanced age. This part is called the hippocampus, a tiny structure in the middle of the brain, which looks a bit like a seahorse, hence its reference to the fish genus bearing the Latin name hippocampus. Of course, we have two hippocampi, one in the right hemisphere and one in the left hemisphere. Each hippocampus has a mean size of well over three cubic centimetres.

The hippocampus is a main player in memory functions, particularly in saving memories for long-term use. To accomplish this important task, the hippocampus can rely on excellent connections. It receives for instance information from the parts of the brain where sensory information is being processed and sends this information along to the parts of the cerebral cortex where intricate cognitive processes take place. When the hippocampus is damaged due to some kind of brain damage, new information can't be stored in long-term memory anymore.

A person who suffers this kind of amnesia, almost immediately loses freshly obtained information. This also concerns for example names and faces. A doctor, who comes to visit the patient, has to introduce himself over and over again.

The hippocampus is one of the parts affected first and most heavily by dementia, caused among others by Alzheimer disease. Alzheimer patients have a substantially smaller hippocampus than healthy people.

Protection

It is of the utmost importance not to expose our indispensable brain to many dangers. Fortunately, Mother Nature has taken a lot of precautionary measures. To begin with, the brain has been wrapped in a very firm skull that can withstand considerable blows.

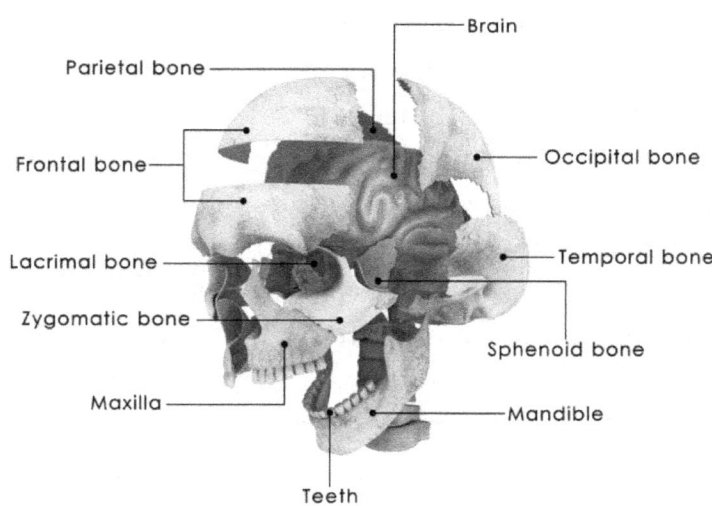

(© 7activestudio - Fotolia.com)

The skull is the brain's first line of defence. It also limits the space available for the brain.

Second in the line of fire are the meninges. They form a flexible, structural, but semipermeable protective pad that completely surrounds the central nervous system. The meninges consist of three membranes.

The dura mater is closest to the skull and surrounds and supports the large venous channels carrying blood from the brain to the heart. The arachnoid mater is the middle membrane, which provides a cushioning effect for the central nervous system. The pia mater firmly adheres to the brain and the spinal cord. The blood vessels going through the pia mater are responsible for nourishing the brain. The meninges are mainly known for the sometimes deadly infection called meningitis.

The next line of defence is the ventricular system. This has two protective functions. It provides an additional structural fluid cushion. It also offers physiological protection via its immunologic functions and its waste disposal system.

The ventricular system is made up of four interconnected cavities: two lateral ventricles, one in the centre of the brain, and one in the brainstem.

The ventricles are filled with fluid, called cerebrospinal fluid. This fluid circulates through the ventricles and around brain and spinal cord. It provides a mechanical cushion to protect the brain from impact with the skull when the head moves. It also allows the brain to float, thus preventing gravity from pushing down the brain upon the lower side of the skull, which would cause serious damage. Cerebrospinal fluid is important in maintaining a constant external environment for brain cells. It takes with it waste from brain metabolism when it enters the blood stream after having circulated. The total volume of cerebrospinal fluid is estimated at 150 millilitres.

Special cells in the ventricular system produce the fluid. This production may lay around 500 millilitres per day.

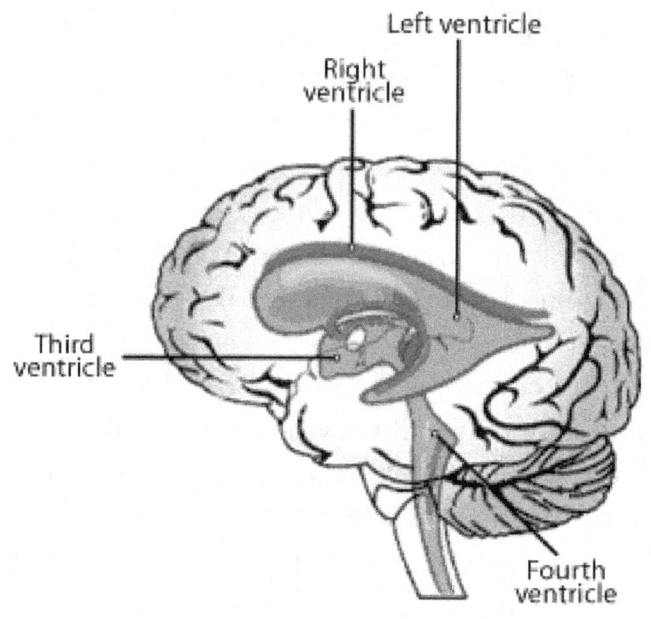

Left ventricle
Right ventricle
Third ventricle
Fourth ventricle

(The brain from top to bottom)

The ventricular system is made up of four interconnected cavities filled with fluid.

The totality of brain mass, blood vessels, and ventricular system has to fit within the available space of our skull. The skull is an absolute, rigid entity. If one part of its contents enlarges another part has to give in. An extension of the totality is not possible. This could lead to problems. An overproduction of cerebrospinal fluid for instance has to be drained via a medical intervention, otherwise brain substance would die.

To make up for changes, the ventricular cavities will expand or contract. The brain shapes the ventricular system. Any changes in the anatomy of the brain can distort the ventricular system and influence ventricle size and shape. When for instance the brain mass deteriorates the ventricles enlarge to fill in the void. Thus the size of the ventricles can be an indicator of the brain's status. Ventricle volumes are extremely diverse between individuals. In general, the ventricles tend to slowly become bigger during ageing. In men, this process starts as of their 40s, in women as of their 50s.

Blood

An adequate blood supply is vital for the brain. Too much blood in our head will raise blood pressure and may cause damage to brain cells, but too little blood could also cause the death of brain cells. Although our brain generally comprises only two percent of our total body weight, it sucks up twenty percent of blood supply, which the heart is pumping around. Blood brings oxygen and nutrients to the brain and takes away waste produced during metabolism in the brain.

The regulation of the blood flow is sensitive down almost to the level of single neurones. It is a complex train of events involving among other things vascular cells and neurones. Blood flow to the brain is tightly coupled with the metabolic demand of local neurones. An increase in neuronal activity leads to an increase in regional cerebral blood flow. Almost instant adjustments are possible. Since neurones are doing overtime, they need extra blood for the delivery of nutrients and for the removal of garbage.

Scientists made clever use of this fact. In the seventies, they started developing equipment to look into the brain-at-work using changes in blood flow. Until that moment, in humans it was only possible to measure electrical activity in the brain. This can be done via electrodes placed on the scalp. The fluctuations in current as registered on a recording device result in an electroencephalogram (EEG). Looking at the produced wave pattern, a specialist can see whether the person's brain activity is within the limits of what has been established as 'normal'. Profound brain research in the past could only be done on animal brains or on donated brains of deceased persons.

Nowadays, with the sophisticated equipment available scientists can scan live human brains. Many people already are familiar with concepts like PET and fMRI. They are abbreviations for complex names of wonderful machines that register blood flow in the brain. When a group of brain cells is activated and more blood flows to that part of the brain, it will show up on such a scan. Thanks to these scans, in a short period our knowledge of the brain has grown exceptionally. Researchers make volunteers carry out certain mental tasks while they are inside the scanner. The scans show the parts of the brain where more blood flows to due to extra activity. Thus certain parts of the brain can be linked to certain mental tasks.

Over the past decades, scientists have scanned the brains of many healthy volunteers. This way, they have gotten a clear picture of what a healthy brain should look like on a scan. By comparing the brain scan of a person with a medical problem with the scans of healthy people, doctors are able to ascertain in which part of the brain something is wrong and what might be the cause of patient's complaints. The resulting diagnosis is far more precise than with the old method, in which the doctor on the basis of questionnaires tries to find out from which part of the brain someone's problems are likely to arise.

Barrier

Our heart pumps blood through our entire body. The blood that flows through our brain has also been in other parts of our body. Therefore it is not only good things the blood might bring to our brain. Harmful substances end up in our blood via for instance our food or the air we breathe in. Generally, our immune system is perfectly capable to put these intruders out of action. But in our brain, many of these substances would cause havoc. So it is a matter of life and death these particles don't reach the brain.

To counteract unwanted intrusion into the brain the blood-brain barrier came into being. This barrier makes sure the brain is well-separated from the rest of our body. Special cells let blood and its useful contents pass, but filter out any other substances. Thus the blood-brain barrier maintains a stable environment for neurones to function effectively.

The blood-brain barrier protects the brain this way, but at the same time is a hurdle medical science has to take. That's because the well-functioning barrier also bans substances doctors would love to see entering the brain. Pharmaceuticals that have been developed specifically to help cure brain diseases usually can't pass the blood-brain barrier either. For example, one of the problems of Parkinson disease is that the brain produces too little dopamine, a substance that activates certain brain cells. An injection of dopamine would then of course be very useful. Unfortunately, this injected dopamine is blocked by the blood-brain barrier and doesn't reach the place where it would be needed. Clever biologists discovered that another substance, levodopa, is able to pass through the blood-brain barrier. Levodopa is the raw material for dopamine. So, when someone is taking pills containing levodopa, this substance will reach the brain and on the spot is being turned into dopamine.

Conquering the blood-brain barrier is one of the biggest challenges for researchers developing drugs for neurological diseases. The barrier is a significant obstacle to drug therapy since the influence of chemical substances depends on how easily they pass through the barrier. Researchers have high expectations of nanotechnology. This technique is directed toward the fabrication of minuscule particles called nano-particles. These particles might be suitable to function as tiny vehicles to help transfer drugs across the blood-brain barrier and deliver the healing substances exactly to the desired spot.

2. INTIMATE RELATIONSHIPS

How do brain cells function?

We all do it every day: to see, to hear, to smell, to move. Most of the time, these activities happen even automatically, without thinking about them. Our brains make sure signals from the outside world are being received. Specialised areas of the brain process the incoming signals. All this information merges in the frontal lobes, the most forward part of the brain. The frontal lobes then send out signals to the inner world of our body. This leads for instance to the fact that we turn our head in the direction of some noise or that we lift our foot when we appear to have reached a staircase we have to climb. All those signals go back and forth in only a fraction of a second. Within this same fraction of a second, the frontal lobes have considered all the possible actions to take and have made a decision about which action would be best suited. How is this possible?

The brain contains two kinds of cells: nerve cells, better known as neurones, and glial cells. Every human brain is made up of an estimated one hundred billion neurones. The number of glial cells is far bigger, about six- to ten-fold.

Up until very recently – and even now still sometimes -, all attention and research efforts went to the neurones. At the beginning of the 20th century, scientists had concluded neurones are the most important brain cells. By that time, new tissue staining techniques had just been developed with which brain tissue could be investigated.

Cells of the Central Nervous System

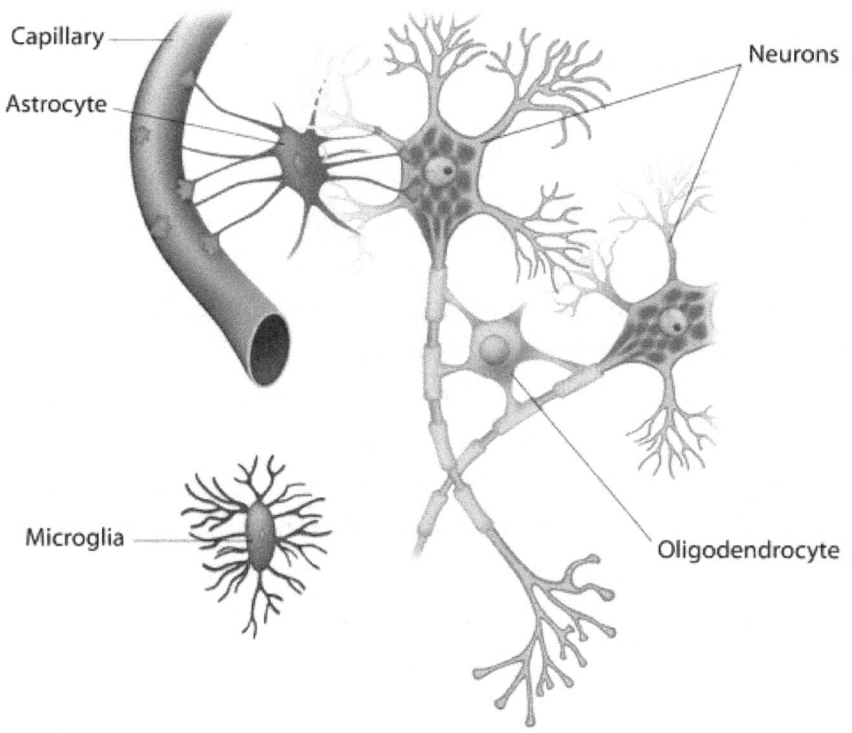

Capillary

Astrocyte

Neurons

Microglia

Oligodendrocyte

(© Alila Medical Media)

Although neurones are better known, glial cells – astrocytes, oligodendrocytes, and microglia - are far more numerous in the human central nervous system.

In the laboratory, a specially prepared slice of brain tissue was injected with a chemical solution containing silver. This solution reacted with individual neurones in the brain slice. These neurones became clearly stained in brown and black and thus stood out in their entirety from the brain pulp.

Today, these and similar staining methods are still being used in laboratories all over the world.

With the limited research methods available at that time, glial cells appeared to do hardly anything. It seemed they only filled up the empty space between neurones. That's why they were named glia, which is Greek for glue. This idea is where the popular belief came from that we only use ten percent of our brain, namely the part that is made up of neurones. Nothing is more beside the truth. Nature doesn't let things just come into being; everything that has no use will disappear in the course of evolution. Hence, it is a bit unreasonable to presume our brains come with a ninety percent reserve capacity.

Later research made perfectly clear most of us use our brains completely, the total one hundred percent. The glial cells have very important tasks in the functioning of the brain as well. The latest research gradually even points to the possibility glia are the most important brain cells. They may be the ones that direct neurones. In Petri dishes (shallow glass or plastic dishes used to culture cells named after their inventor, the German bacteriologist Julius Richard Petri) in the laboratory, glial cells are able to survive on their own whereas neurones will only stay alive in the dish when they are accompanied by glia.

Information

The picture we have of the functioning of the different brain cells is getting clearer now. This is thanks to new research methods and ever smaller and more sensitive measuring equipment that becomes available. In the laboratory, it is even possible at present to attach tiny measuring devices to one single neurone. This is nothing short of a miracle; considering the fact neurones averagely have a diameter of about twenty micrometer (one micrometer is one-thousandth of a millimeter).

Many different types of neurones exist. The most common type consists of a nucleus, a long sprout on one side, called axon, and one or more short sprouts with several branches on the other side. These little fingers are called dendrites. Neurones are champions in information transfer. Via their dendrites, they catch a signal from another neurone or from a glial cell. This signal is processed within the neurone, which results in another signal being sent out via the other side of the neurone, via the axon. The next neurone in the chain subsequently catches and processes the signal, and so forth.

Human Neuron Anatomy

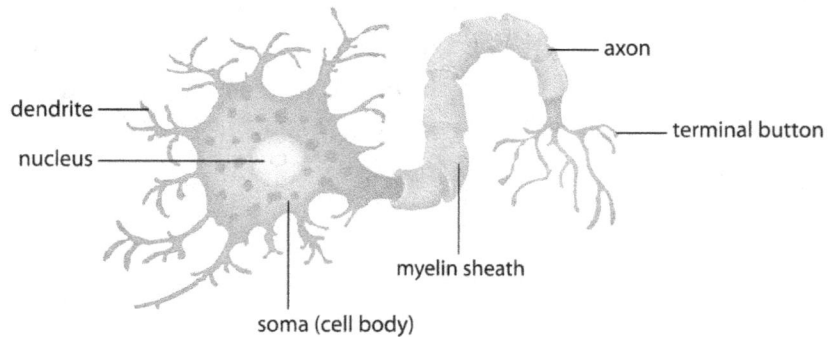

(© blueringmedia - Fotolia.com)

The most common type of neurone consists of an axon on one side to send out signals and dendrites on the other side to receive signals.

The transfer of information is made up of small electric currents. These impulses pass relatively slow through the neurone, varying from 1 to at most 120 meters per second. For comparison: the cruise speed of a Boeing 747 passenger jet is 250 meters per second.

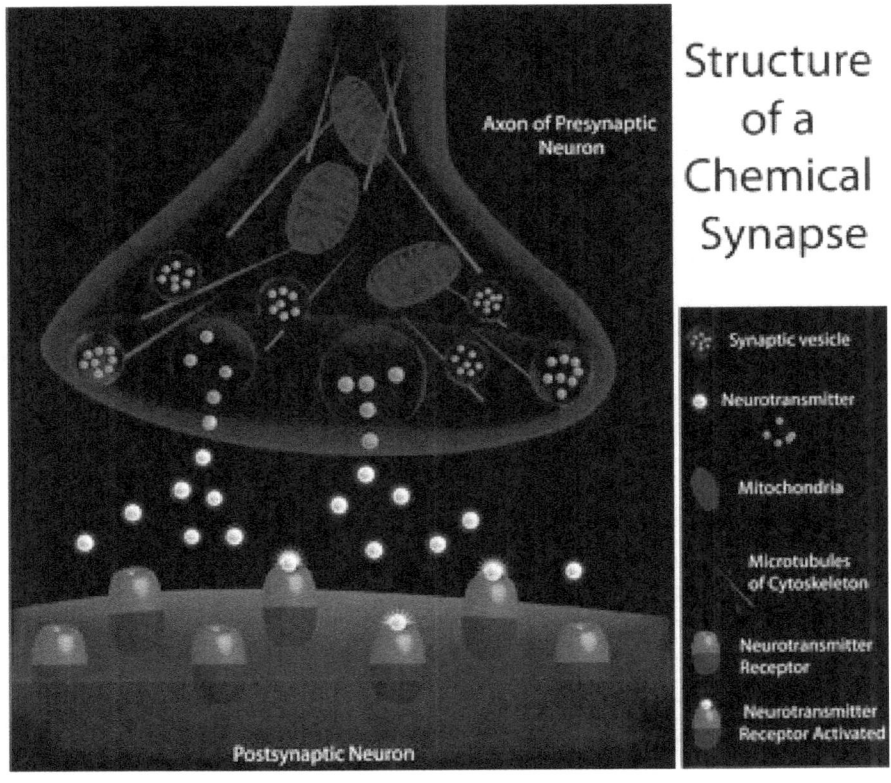

Structure of a Chemical Synapse

Axon of Presynaptic Neuron

Synaptic vesicle

Neurotransmitter

Mitochondria

Microtubules of Cytoskeleton

Neurotransmitter Receptor

Neurotransmitter Receptor Activated

Postsynaptic Neuron

(© Alila Medical Media)

Neurones generally don't make physical contact. They send and receive chemical substances called neurotransmitters to communicate.

In general, neurones don't make physical contact with each other. There's a minute opening between the axon of one neurone and the receiving dendrite of the next neurone, called the synapse.

Every time the electric current in the neurone reaches the end of the axon, it spits out a chemical substance. This substance crosses the synapse and sticks to one of the dendrites of the neurone on the other side. The chemical reaction this causes brings into being another electric current that travels through the neurone. This process repeats itself infinite times.

The chemical substance a neurone spits out via its axon is called neurotransmitter. Many types of neurotransmitters have already been discovered, but it is very likely more substances exist that function as neurotransmitter and that haven't been discovered yet.

Normally, neurones specialise and produce only one type of neurotransmitter.

Some well-known names of neurotransmitters are serotonin, acetylcholine, glutamate, and GABA. Every neurotransmitter has its own tasks within the nervous system. Serotonin, for example, stimulates neurones involved in learning and memory, but also neurones that regulate our mood. A shortage of serotonin appears to play a role in depression.

Dopamine is the neurotransmitter of the reward circuit in our brain. When we do something we like, a lot of dopamine is released and that makes us feel good. As a consequence, we start doing that enjoyable thing more often. This is how nature makes sure we keep on doing things that are useful for our survival and reproduction.

Nature hasn't kept up with modern times though. Nowadays, the reward system isn't always promoting useful behaviour.

We do things we like very much and that activate dopamine release, but that are very damaging to our health and survival, like eating too much fat and practicing extreme sports. A shortage of dopamine is pinpointed in Parkinson disease. Errors in the dopamine system have also been found in people who suffer schizophrenia.

Acetylcholine among other things takes care of information transfer to the muscles. Glutamate is the most common neurotransmitter and is involved in learning and memory. GABA is the chief inhibitory neurotransmitter. It regulates neuronal excitability.

Networking

One neurone communicates with on average about seven thousand other neurones. These contacts are variable. Depending on requirement, a neurone at one time communicates with this neighbour and at another time with that one. The better it knows its neighbour the easier it starts talking to her. Contacts with new neighbours or neighbours it hasn't spoken to for a long time are harder.

In some people, neurones have too many connections. They suffer from a condition called synaesthesia, in which stimulation of one sense also arouses sensation in another. This sensory phenomenon results in cross-sense experiences, such as colour-hearing, colour-tasting, taste-hearing, and smell-vision. Grapheme-colour synaesthesia, in which an individual's perception of numbers and letters is associated with the experience of colours, is the most common form of the condition.

Synaesthesia has to do with the abnormal merging of neural networks. In the baby brain, a mishmash of connections is still quite common. The brain of a newly born isn't ready yet. The basic architecture with all its structures is there, but networks are still under development. There's a lot of babbling going on and neurones seem to communicate randomly. During the first months and years in the life of a human being, so much is going on in the brain. As a child grows, establishing new connections and breaking up unused ones thins out, but it is an ongoing process and only by the time a person reaches his thirties all the basic neural networks have formed.

The area of the frontal lobes behind your forehead, called the prefrontal cortex, is the last part to completely come online. It is in this prefrontal cortex your personality and your ability to take responsible decisions are coordinated. Watching the behaviour of teens and people in their twenties, it is often very clear their prefrontal cortex has not yet fully developed. During the growth of a baby in the womb, neurones make contacts in abundance. Stimulated by nutrients present in the brain and not hindered by information from the exterior, the neurones keep on chattering with as many neighbours as they encounter. It is as if they are practicing for the time they will be functioning in the outside world. They end up with far too many, often useless contacts.

After birth, most of these connections will be broken again. Fine-tuning takes place influenced by information that enters the brain from outside. With the maturation of the brain, extensive pruning of axons happens and stronger connections form between the cells in one sensory system, sharpening and separating the senses.

This process continues throughout life, but is going on rather rigorously in the first years of one's existence. Of course from time to time something goes wrong in this fine-tuning process. Connections that should have been broken may continue to exist.

This may be the explanation for synaesthesia. At about three months of age, all children probably are synesthetes. In adults who suffer synaesthesia, the pruning process apparently hasn't been finished completely. Neurones involved in the processing of letters or numbers for example have unusual connections with neurones that are active in the processing of colours. Or neurones from taste networks communicate simultaneously with neurones in sound networks. Synaesthesia is a harmless, but, for the person involved, very interesting abnormality. It used to be considered a very rare condition, but now it has been shown to be rather common, appearing in maybe as much as about 1 in every 200 persons. Synaesthesia runs in families and hence is at least partly genetically induced. The condition is much more common among people in creative professions, like artists and writers. Apparently, creative and abstract thinking is linked to neurones with an above normal number of connections in certain parts of the brain. Famous people known to be synesthetes are among others the composers and musicians Franz Liszt, Duke Ellington, Frank Zappa and Lady Gaga, the Greek mathematician Pythagoras, the actress Marilyn Monroe, and the Russian writer Vladimir Nabokov. But essentially we all have some form of synaesthesia when for example we experience high musical notes as clear and low notes as dark. Or when we feel blue, see red or are green with envy.

Matrix
For the past century, brain science has been dominated by the

neural doctrine. We speak of neuroscience, neurosurgeon, and neurodegeneration.

There even was a time, it was said we only use ten percent of our brains since neurones represent only ten percent of all brain cells. Maybe in the coming decade a revolution will take place as 'the other' brain cell will get its well-deserved attention.

Glial cells have long played only a secondary role in brain science. Due to limited technology, all research efforts focused on the easier to understand neurone. Thanks to big technical advances it is possible now to study glia more in detail in laboratories and the results are surprising. More and more astonishing facts about these brain cells are emerging and it is becoming clear glia are very sophisticated cogs in the brain machinery.

So far, we have learned the brain is made up of an incredibly complicated web of neurones. Glial cells are responsible for organising this tangle of excitable cells and give an efficient structure to the brain. They play a key part in orchestrating neuronal functioning and survival.

Different types of glia exist. The most common is called astrocyte. Collectively, these astrocytes form a kind of matrix in our brain. Every astrocyte controls and manages its own little piece of brain, including neurones and neurotransmitters present. When a problem arises astrocytes step in, for instance by closing off the damaged part from the rest of the brain. Sometimes astrocytes overdo it. They go haywire, grow explosively and become a brain tumour.

To be able to accomplish all their tasks, astrocytes are assisted by another type of glial cells, the microglia. These cells make up the immune system of the brain. They constantly scan their domain for intruders. The moment they encounter one, they will attack the alien cell and destroy it.

The third type of glial cell is of crucial importance for a well-functioning brain. It is the oligodendrocyte, a puzzling Greek word that means 'cell with a few branches'. This glial cell enwraps the axons of neurones with a fatty, white substance, called myelin. This sheath enables better conductivity within the axon so as to make the electric currents reach the tip faster. You can compare its working with the plastic wrapping around an electricity cable.

MULTIPLE SCLEROSIS

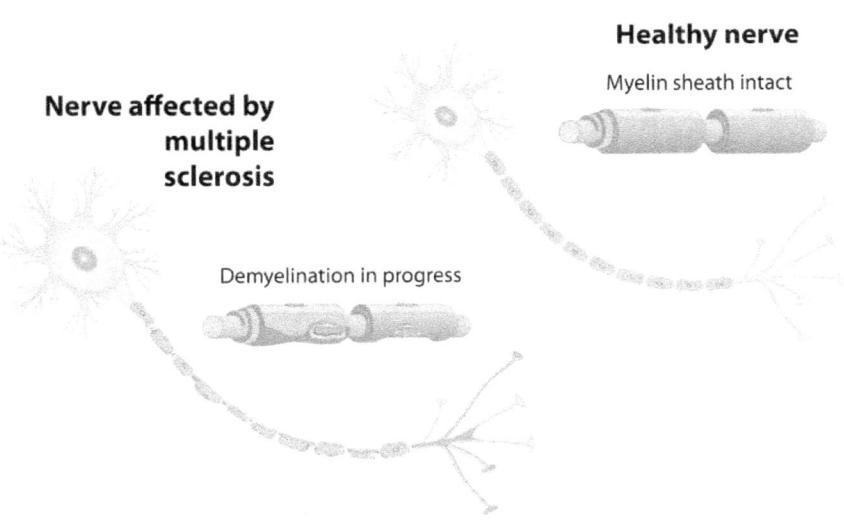

Healthy nerve

Myelin sheath intact

Nerve affected by multiple sclerosis

Demyelination in progress

(© designua - Fotolia.com)

Multiple sclerosis affects the myelin sheath surrounding the neurone's axon and thus disrupts communication.

In various diseases, of which multiple sclerosis is best known, this fatty sheath is being affected and gradually disappears. The electric currents won't pass through the axons anymore and information transfer becomes blocked.

It is clear glia are extremely important for the well-being of the brain. They are involved in just about all diseases in the brain, for better or for worse. The reactions of glial cells are of critical importance to the process of a neural pathology.

Most drugs that have been developed so far though aim at neurones and specifically neurotransmitters. Future research has to come up with remedies to help glial cells continue to do their good work.

Through the ages, scientists have been intrigued by the intellectual capabilities of the human being in comparison to those of other animals.

What makes one animal more intelligent than another? The size of the brain cannot be decisive since there are many animals with bigger brains than humans. And even the brains of the Neanderthals were larger than those of modern man. Neurones don't vary that much either. In comparison with neurones of rats and mice for instance those of humans are only a bit longer.

The rise in intelligence does coincide with the number of glia. The brains of animals that are higher up on the intelligence ladder hold more glial cells per neurone. Astrocytes in human brains have proven to be bigger, faster and more complex than those in the brains of other animals.

It might just be we owe our bigger brainpower to the fact that our astrocytes are more sophisticated and have more complex processing abilities.

It has been shown the brain of the famous physics genius

Albert Einstein which was preserved after his death, contained far more glia than the brains of ordinary men to which it was compared.

3. ONCE UPON A TIME

What are memories?

We have seen so far, the electric currents that jump from neurone to neurone cause a lot of actions in our body. They make us do, see, and feel all kinds of things. But we don't do, see, and feel the same every day, every month, and every year. We also evolve. We learn to walk, talk, read, write, ride a bicycle, drive a car, and many, many more things. We remember how to do certain things and we remember where we've been on holiday ten years ago. How do we do that? The brains of all living organisms have one very peculiar trait. They can learn and remember. Learning is about gaining knowledge of the world in which the organism lives. Memory is responsible for safeguarding this knowledge and making it accessible whenever necessary.
It is clearly of great advantage if an animal is good at learning and remembering. To know that a certain watering hole should be avoided because of all the predators that come to drink there is very useful for survival.
The same goes true for the ability to remember where one can find certain foods. Animals that perform well as far as learning and remembering are concerned stay alive for a longer period. They procreate more and generally their offspring will inherit the useful traits of father and mother. Evolution cherishes learning and memory capabilities this way.
Learning is an ongoing, lifelong process. Every time

something is learned, a tiny change takes place in the brain. This in turn helps to learn something new. The learning depends on the environment in which a specific animal has been living. Animals are biologically programmed to learn specific things, to learn to fear specific objects for instance. They don't learn behaviours outside of their evolutionary adaptation. The sea slug has no need for mathematics, but being able to release clouds of ink to blind an attacker does come in handy. The faster its neurones respond, the better its defence is. The nervous systems, which come in a huge variety, are built to accomplish certain tasks. Learning helps to do the job better.

The human brain isn't a general-purpose device which can be trained to do almost anything. It comes with a specific organisation to allow for specific responses to specific challenges. The knowledge we acquire also results from interactions with the environment. Knowledge stacks up like building blocks. If you have mastered the art of talking, afterwards you can easily learn how to sing, although not always in tune. If you have mastered the art of getting hold of something, subsequently you can learn how to knit or how to build something without a huge effort.

Links

Everything our brain contains, so everything we know and do, can be brought back to contacts between neurones and glial cells. The many billions of brain cells all have their specific tasks and form specialised networks. Whenever we learn something new, another network is created. All neurones that have been involved in for instance performing a certain activity have created an invisible bond. One neurone has communicated with another one, its neighbour. At first, they only greeted from a distance. But now that they know each other, next time they meet they will have a casual chat across the hedge. If they see each other often enough there even may result a shortcut through the hedge so they can easily visit each other for a cup of coffee.

Close-knit networks of neurones that frequently communicate with each other are being established this way. The contacts one neurone makes with other neurones are not fixed. They can change constantly. Depending on necessity a cell is in contact with one cell one moment and with another cell another moment. This all is influenced by what you are doing, what you are thinking, what is going on around you. Contacts come and go. Cells that have to communicate regularly gain very strong links that normally won't be broken anymore. This is the case for example for cells that have to be active when you are walking.

Contacts made during a one-off activity or for something you have learned a long time ago, may be lost if the connections aren't used anymore. That is why it is so hard to remember certain difficult things you learned at school, unless they have been hammered into your brain like some historical facts which you can sum up immediately. The network made at that time is so secure it is almost impossible to untie.

That is for instance also the case in a post-traumatic stress disorder. This is a severe anxiety disorder that can develop after exposure to a very traumatic event. A person that has been in a life threatening situation can still suffer nightmares, increased arousal, and other mental problems many years later. The network that was created during the traumatic event can hardly be dissolved anymore and many therapy sessions at a psychologist are necessary to make the fear and distress manageable.

What the psychologist is trying to do together with the patient is close off the shortcuts through the hedge that automatically bring up the fearful images. Instead the neurones involved have to make contact with other neighbours so that together they will conjure a more objective picture of the traumatic event. This may be brought about by recounting the story over and over again and realising the experience admittedly was awful, but not the end of the world. During this learning process neurones involved establish new connections and bit by bit the old, undesired network becomes obsolete.

How can a dramatic experience become so intensely engraved in your memory? This has to do with the amygdala, almond-shaped clusters of neurones deep within the temporal lobes of both hemispheres. The amygdala is in charge of the emotional side of memories. It is activated when an experience has an emotional load. The more intense the emotion the more ineradicable the memory becomes.

Classification

In the past decades, a lot of time and money has been spent to study human memory. Despite all this effort, we still don't know exactly how our memory functions. Clearly, it is very difficult to reduce recollections of your father who passed away or of your first love to electric currents in your brain and brain cells forming networks.

The man, who made the biggest progress in our knowledge of how memory works, is the American scientist Eric Kandel. For his pioneering research he earned himself a Nobel Prize. A tiny creature assisted Kandel in his studies: a sea slug named

Aplysia. This slug has a very simple nervous system with only a few thousand, relatively large neurones. Notwithstanding this simplicity, Aplysia is able to learn and form memories. Hence, an excellent organism to lend a hand in the discovery of the basic principles of memory.

Lately, memory research has deepened even further thanks to our knowledge of genes that has been gathered in the past decades. Genes hold the hereditary material of an organism. Scientists nowadays are able to alter mice genetically. They can either introduce a new gene (transgene) into a mouse brain or delete a specific, existing gene (knockout). This way, they can research which genes are involved in the process of learning and the formation of memories and what their tasks are. Thanks to new and ever more sophisticated imaging techniques it is now also possible to study live human brains while exercising learning and memory tasks.

Although we normally use the word memory, it isn't just one entity. It is an umbrella concept. In practice, several types of memory have been classified. Of course this is a classification we humans have made. Within the various schools of psychology, different classifications of memory are being used. Clearly, all this variability does not help comprehensibility of a topic of which we aren't completely in the know anyway.

The scholars do agree on the fact that we have sensory memory. This is the recording of what we perceive with our senses. It is very short-lived and lasts from milliseconds to seconds. Sensory memory functions outside of our consciousness. We are not aware it exists and don't have access to the information it contains. Needless to say, the brain does use this sensory information without us knowing it.

You are able, for example, to dodge a stone that was thrown at you unexpectedly before you became conscious of the fact that a stone was coming towards you. The brain receives an image via your eyes and immediately sends signals directly to your muscles. As a result, your body makes a movement to elude the stone that is approaching rapidly without you having started any action.

Our short-term memory we use to keep some information for a short period, such as a telephone number. It has a lifetime of seconds to minutes and can only hold in general about seven plus or minus two items. We are consciously aware of the contents of short-term memory. Information automatically disappears from short-term memory, often because it has been replaced by something else we want to remember for a moment. If the information is important to us and we repeat it several times it may transfer to long-term memory.

Working memory is a broadening and deepening of the simple short-term memory. It is a limited-capacity store for maintenance and manipulation. It retains information over the short-term and it performs mental operations on its contents. This information comes from sensory memory and from long-term memory. An example: you walk in a street and from a window in one of the houses along the street a delicious smell of food enters your nostrils. You activate your working memory to think about which dish could belong to this delicious smell and to search in your long-term memory to find out when was the last time you ate this dish.

Information that has reached long-term memory will stay there for days, years or even a lifetime. Long-term memory contains two types of memory: non-declarative and declarative memory.

Non-declarative memory is about knowledge to which we have no conscious access. It contains among other things skills we have learned. When we learn to ride a bicycle for instance, at first it is very difficult and we have to put a lot of effort and all our attention into it. After a while, we cycle more or less automatically and don't think about it anymore while we are doing it. Our cycling skill has been engraved in the unconscious part of long-term memory.

Declarative memory handles knowledge to which we have conscious access. It comprises information about our own lives and world knowledge we have learned. We can purposely recall these memories. Sometimes, you just can't find what you are looking for, possibly because you are tired. In other circumstances, mainly because of diseases like Alzheimer disease, someone won't be able to retrieve memories at all anymore, because the brain has been damaged and the cellular network of a memory has fallen apart.

Reconstruction

Our memories are extremely valuable. They make us who we are. Memories are a prerequisite for feeling human. Severely impaired memory deprives people of a sense of personal continuity. It isolates them from emotionally or practically meaningful contact with the world around and renders them passive and dependent. Even mildly to moderately impaired memory has a disorienting effect. Someone who doesn't have memories anymore has lost himself.

Notwithstanding their exceptional worth, even all those beautiful, sad, pleasant, and annoying memories again can be reduced to electric currents in our brains. An efficient memory system requires intact functioning of many brain regions.

It is not known yet exactly how memories are stored in the brain, but bit by bit an interesting image has come up how this process most likely is taking place. It is absolutely certain the brain does not record memories like some kind of photographs or videotapes and afterwards when the memories are being recalled, shows them on a type of screen in one's head.

Widespread brain areas cooperate in learning and memory. Individual structures form systems for specific memory processes. Memories are stored in those parts of the brain that were involved when the information entered the brain in the first place.

When you think of your grandmother you see her face, smell her perfume, feel her cheek that you used to kiss, and hear her voice. All that information entered during encounters with your grandmother in different parts of your brain, dedicated to your eyes, your nose, your skin, and your ears.

Many years later, when your grandmother has long passed away and you recall the cherished memory of her, the information from those different parts of your brain comes together in your working memory to make you see, smell, feel, and hear that familiar image of granny.

Hippocampus

The hippocampus is a key player in memory. This tiny group of brain cells sits like a spider on the web of incoming and potentially preserved information. Scientists have been able to study the functions of the hippocampus in mice. They damaged the hippocampi of specially bred mice and watched what would be the consequences.

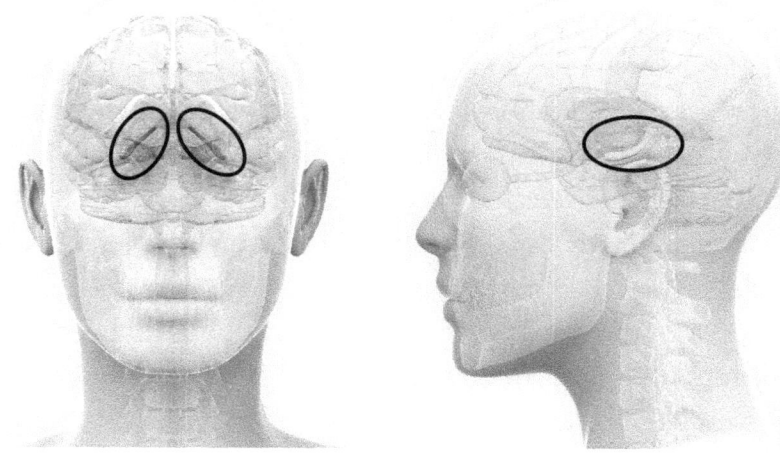

A tiny group of brain cells called hippocampus (circled) is a key player in memory. The hippocampus needs special care as it is very vulnerable to the ageing process.

Many research projects have yielded proof that the hippocampus is critical for forming new long-term memories. It may be a temporary way station for information to enter long-term memory. As the parts of a memory are stored in the areas of the brain that initially processed the information, the hippocampus may serve to bind together the various components of a memory. If desired, the amygdala adds an emotional touch to the memory, for instance the happy feeling you had when you were going to visit your grandmother. Memories can also be deceiving. That is due to the fact that a memory is the reconstruction of facts and experiences as they are stored in your brain. It is not a reconstruction of what actually happened. Just ask a policeman about the many problems they always have with eyewitness reports. Ten people have seen exactly the same event, but every one of them gives a different description of what happened. This is caused not only by the fact that one person pays attention to other details than another person, but above all because the brain gives its own interpretation to the facts. You are looking at an event with your brain and your brain differs from the brain of everybody else. Your brain contains networks that coincide with experiences you had so far in your life.

This causes an event to be stored in memory in a somewhat biased way. The situation becomes even more difficult during recollection of the memory. Recall isn't an exact copy of the information originally stored, as the brain reconstructs a past event. The result is a memory of an event that already has been interpreted twice.

Every time a memory is recalled and subsequently put back into storage a possibility of changes exists. The more time has gone by between the saving of the original memory and its recall, the greater the chance of modifications. Besides, the brain that is retrieving the memory from storage isn't the same brain anymore that put it there. Networks come and go. Our brain is in constant movement because of everything we learn and experience.

Specialisation

Learning is based on alterations in connections between neurones. Whenever these changes are permanent a memory is formed.

Every time we learn something new, connections between neurones come into being. To be able to perform the new task neurones with different specialisations are being recruited, for instance from the visual or the motor areas of the brain. This specialisation of neurones goes really far.

A good example is the way our vision is organised. The visual cortex is the most intensely investigated part of the brain so far. When we look at a certain object, one neurone in the visual areas is activated when we see a vertical straight line and other neurones are activated by seeing a horizontal straight line or by a diagonal line or by an arched line. In short, many, many specialised neurones are active to make us see a complete image.

For each task, another network of neurones is activated, but each neurone takes part in several networks and is thus involved in different tasks, be it with different partners.

The more often a new task is being repeated, the smoother contacts between neurones involved will come about. This is due to the fact that a larger quantity of neurotransmitter, the chemical substance that transfers signals from one neurone to the next, becomes ready for use. The other brain cells, the glial cells, play an important part in this process as well. Besides, the receiving neurone grows more dendrites on which receptors are available for the extra neurotransmitter molecules. All this contributes to an even better information transfer.

As a result, connections between those neurones are less volatile. Information isn't that easily forgotten anymore and passes from short-term memory to long-term memory. These names are made up by us humans. It doesn't mean information actually goes to another place in the brain. The neurones involved have developed due to which they changed jobs and they are now working as part of long-term memory.

Memory

Poor Memory

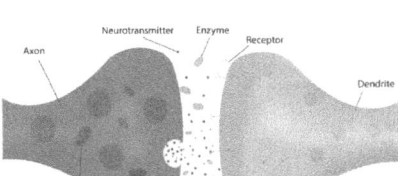

Good Memory

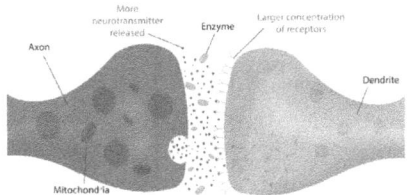

(© joshya – Fotolia.com)

Connections between neurones form the basics of memory. The more effective neurones communicate the more stable a memory is.

Sleep appears to play an important role in this process of information transferring from short-term to long-term memory.

The network that had been activated while we were learning something new is again being activated when we take a rest. The brain replays the process of information transfer concerned so that the neurones involved know they are participants in that specific network. In other words, the contacts between various neighbours become more intimate. When we sleep no new information from the outside world enters the brain. This is the most perfect moment for the brain to do some serious cleaning up!

The hippocampus sends the newly made memories to the various brain areas concerned. There the above-mentioned changes take place in the amount of neurotransmitter and the number of receptors. Thanks to these changes, the memories become part of long-term memory.

Forgetting

Not everything we experience and learn ends up in long-term memory. It would be disastrous if that would be the case. Total recall would paralyse us mentally. Some examples are known of people who are able to remember everything they did in their lives since they were young, a disorder called hyperthymesia. This is a life-disrupting disorder since sufferers cannot control the constant stream of memories. Forgetting is a perfectly normal, everyday experience and a positive one. Efficient memory means we forget much of what we experience, far more than we remember. Memory tends to be best for meaningful and important matters. For example, you normally don't remember what you have eaten three days ago. These facts are so irrelevant they are not preserved. Evolution shaped memory to mainly store information we might need.

Some annoying or painful memories that have been stored efficiently you would prefer to forget. The more you try to forget them, the better they become engraved in long-term memory since you are activating the networks concerned over and over again. Often time lends a helping hand because a network becomes less firm over time. Forming new memories is also very useful because then other, older memories will disappear into the background.

Of course it would be fantastic if you could erase just one, nasty memory by taking a pill. We still have some time to go before such a remedy will exist, but scientists have made good progress in understanding what happens in and between brain cells during the process of forgetting. They have discovered a protein that is in particular involved in fearful memories. An overdose of this protein can erase these scary memories. In their laboratory, the researchers have succeeded in deleting just one specific scary memory in mice. People will have to wait a little longer before they can make use of this technique since it involves manipulation of genes and it is still unclear what would be the consequences of that.

4. WHO AM I ?

Research into consciousness

The state of being conscious constitutes the final taboo in brain research. How can it be that I feel like me and that I can think about myself? For many decades, this topic had been hiding deep inside the drawers of scientists in brain laboratories. Our culture and most of all religions had made consciousness a controversial theme. For centuries, people have been raised with the idea they have a soul and that this soul after their deaths will live forever in some kind of hereafter.

Even for many people working with the brain, like psychiatrists and psychologists and indeed some neuroscientists, it is very hard to cope with the fact that everything we do and know, all our problems and happy moments, would derive from activated networks in the brain. There has to be something else since everybody has a very strong sense of self. The general idea is, this ego, as it is also referred to, has to come from somewhere and has to dwell in some place.

Fortunately, a policy change is gradually coming about. Interest in serious scientific research into consciousness is growing.

The thing that complicates this kind of investigation the most is precisely this consciousness itself. Our self is only too eager to have us believe it is very important and extraordinary. It is not easy to step outside of yourself, take some distance and think realistically about that person inside your head.

For centuries, philosophers have been looking for the seat of our soul. The stomach and the heart have long been the favourite places for the soul's residence.

Also in the brain, diligent searches have been going on to find the spot that would contain our self. But this research didn't bring in any results.

Of course, since there is no such place inside our brain that holds our ego. Everything we are and think, all our convictions and ideas are products of brain cells making connections.

"I think, therefore I am", assumed the French philosopher René Descartes at the beginning of the 17th century. With this statement he laid the foundation of the separation between body and mind which has dominated our thinking for centuries and in many cases still does so.

The assertion in fact should be "I am, therefore I think", because our thoughts arise from physical brain activity. The philosopher Baruch Spinoza, born in Amsterdam from Portuguese parents and living in about the same time as Descartes, already had figured this out. In one of his works, titled Ethica and published in 1677, he positioned that the human mind is the idea of the human body.

Mirror

Consciousness is a somewhat elusive concept. We know we are conscious, but what about other animals? An ape or a dog cannot tell us they are endowed with a sense of self. Initially, it was presumed only human beings possessed consciousness. A clear example of the arrogance of mankind to always feel superior to all other living beings! Slowly, man became more sober-minded and scientists found signals probably more animal species have some form of consciousness.

A means to find out whether this is true is the mirror test. Do animal species other than humans recognise themselves in the mirror? To perform the test, a stain is applied to the animal's skin. When the animal sees itself in the mirror and touches the stain on its skin or tries to rub it away it is clear the animal knows the mirror image is his. To make the test watertight, a similar stain, but made from invisible material, is applied to another part of the animal's skin so as to make sure it is not the sensation of the stain that makes the animal investigate or remove the visible stain.

Children as of one and a half years of age, successfully come through the test. But the other members of the hominidae or great apes, namely gorillas, orang-utans, and chimpanzees, also don't have difficulty at all to recognise themselves in the mirror. Even dolphins, pigeons, elephants, and magpies have passed the mirror test with flying colours.

Apparently there are more animals with at least a rudimentary form of consciousness. Up to what grade their consciousness works we don't know yet. Is a pigeon on some windowsill not only thinking about food, but also contemplating its existence and its place in the world? We will only be able to find that out when we would have encountered the networks in the brain that are activated when our ego comes online. Only then can we find out whether similar networks are being activated in the brains of other animals.

Consciousness is one of our brain's functions. Therefore it should be possible to decipher the biological mechanisms within the brain that give rise to consciousness. It is evident a brain activity should persist for some time to pop up in consciousness. It is also clear we only become aware of brain activities that reach our frontal lobes, responsible for our superior thought processes.

Scientists have different ideas about why one activity in the brain does reach consciousness and another activity does not. Most of them do agree on one thing. Conscious experiences are not caused by specific parts of the brain. Consciousness is brought into being foremost by processes, by the exchange of information between brain cells.

For the most part, traffic between the different levels within the brain is one-way. Information enters via the senses, reaches intermediate distribution centres in different parts of the brain, and from there goes up to the frontal lobes. In the frontal lobes, adequate action is formulated, for which subsequently information is sent down the chain, all the way to the corresponding body part. Consciousness might possibly be the result of the fact that certain information is not transferred immediately, but keeps reverberating for a while in the networks. Via a kind of short-term memory we might become aware of this information.

A new theory of consciousness concerns astrocytes, the most numerous glial cells in the brain. They may form the biological basis for our consciousness. Earlier we saw these astrocytes make up a sort of matrix in the brain. They are intertwined. One astrocyte makes contact this way with as much as fifty to one hundred other astrocytes in its vicinity. All those astrocytes communicate with each other via calcium currents. They also direct neurones via calcium injections.

The chemical element calcium is indispensable for all forms of life on earth. It is not only necessary for the structure of bones, but plays a crucial role in the functioning of cells as well. The fact that astrocytes govern the quantity of calcium in the brain, gives some clue about how important these brain cells are.

It might be the calcium waves that flow through the astrocyte matrix that give rise to our consciousness. This idea isn't so far-fetched, especially considering the fact that the number of astrocytes per neurone in a brain becomes larger as animals reach higher stages of development. Besides, the astrocyte is the most common brain cell in the human cortex. It seems the number of astrocytes is coupled to brainpower. More astrocytes appear to give rise to a larger capacity of complex cognitive processes.

Unconscious

How brain generates consciousness and what actually is the biological basis of it, time will tell. It is a fact that the greatest part of what is going on in our brain happens outside of consciousness. Nobody has to consciously think about making sure their heart is beating, their stomach is digesting the food it contains, or their thyroid gland is producing the necessary hormones. Many of our thought processes even develop unconsciously. Don't we all have the experience that often at the least expected moment, for instance when in bed or while walking in the supermarket, suddenly the solution to a problem occurs to you and you were absolutely not thinking of the problem at that moment. Often, a decision has already been taken by your unconscious brain long before your consciousness gets hold of what is going on and announces it has come up with a decision.

It is very fortunate many things we do, proceed automatically.

If we would have to think about every action we take it would be very time-consuming. It could even be life-threatening. In a dangerous situation, your brain has to be able to immediately prepare your body for fight or flight. Your consciousness would only be in the way in such circumstances.

Artists and top athletes know all about the sometimes obstructing influence of consciousness. When they let their self have its say it negatively influences their performance. It will make them consciously think about what they are doing when they actually should lose themselves in their intuition. In these kinds of activities, the best achievements result when the brain is left to doing its thing without interruption.

Aberrations

Why do we possess consciousness? At a certain time in evolution, consciousness may have arisen as some kind of aberration. Many of the useful adaptations of organisms have once come about this way, as a deviation of the standard, the normal.

For example, at one time a butterfly was born with a specific coloration on its wings that looked like eyes. Birds considered this coloration to be real eyes and thought it dangerous to eat the butterfly. They left it alone. The butterfly led a long and fruitful life, had a lot of offspring who all had the same special coloration on their wings. The descendants also reproduced successfully. Finally, all members of this butterfly type ended up with the abnormality, which proved to be very useful.

Not all aberrations have the same advantageous influence on reproduction. These useless ones will simply disappear as a matter of course. But the beneficial abnormalities will become normality in the course of evolution.

This may very well be the case where consciousness is concerned. It appears to be advantageous for an organism to have a brain with two states: unconscious and conscious. In the unconscious state, the brain takes care of fast, often stereotypical reactions. In the conscious state, processes are far slower, but it helps the brain come up with deliberate reactions to complicated situations. Both states can also influence each other. It seems this division has been useful to survival to such an extent that we now have all been equipped with it.

Thanks to our consciousness, we do everything to survive as long as possible. We worship our ego and when the moment of death eventually has arrived, we desperately cling to the idea that our self will live on forever. The indestructible faith in a life after death may even be considered the most successful aberration of evolution.

But, as British neuroscientist and winner of a Nobel Prize Francis Crick used to say so metaphorically: you are nothing but a pack of neurones.

PART II GENES

By discovering the structure of the DNA molecule, science
made a giant leap forward. For the reader with eye for detail, I
will write down the complete name just once:
deoxyribonucleic acid. But you can immediately forget that
awfully difficult name. Just remember that the DNA molecule
contains our hereditary information, our genetic instructions.
One gene is a little piece of the DNA molecule. One DNA
molecule may contain many genes. In the past decades,
biological science has been dominated by the quest to
decipher the secrets of these genes. The genome of an
organism is its complete package of hereditary information.
At the beginning of the 21st century, scientists had more or
less unravelled the complete human genome. Had they
assumed at first we would have a couple of millions of genes,
in the end it seems the human genome only holds about
20,000 genes.

Aided by this new knowledge of our genes, researchers now
try to discover where certain diseases originate. Nobody is
perfect and everybody has an amount of defects in their
genes. Those defects may cause problems in the functioning of
our body, which can lead to diseases.

Wouldn't it be fantastic if in the future we would know which
defects in which genes may generate which diseases? And it
would be even more tremendous of course if we would be
able to repair those defect genes or replace them.

Frequently, headlines appear in newspapers and magazines
about the discovery of a specific gene that is supposedly the
originator of a certain disease ("New Alzheimer genes

discovered", "Scientists find autism gene"). Most of the time, new knowledge about genes and heredity is published somewhat oversimplified for the general public. The impression is given our genes determine who we are. And more importantly: which diseases we will be suffering from. It seems the genes we inherit from our parents have an inescapable fate in store for us.

Nothing is more besides the truth, as will become clear from the explanation about heredity, genes, and ageing in the coming chapters.

5. EUREKA

What do genes do?

Small, icy rooms without heating and English pubs where a lot of alcohol is flowing are ingredients not only for many exciting detective stories, but also for the story of the discovery of the DNA molecule.

In his book The Double Helix, the American biologist James Watson describes the quest for the structure of DNA. The find was not at all like the happy moment of the Greek philosopher Archimedes who more than two thousand years ago, while sitting in a bath tub, all of a sudden came up with the solution to a physics problem and exclaimed: "Eureka" (I have found it).

On the contrary, it took two years of obsessiveness at the beginning of the fifties in the last century. Watson was working with Francis Crick at the University of Cambridge in England.

Many lunches were dedicated to discussions about the structure of DNA. Ideas cropped up and could then be thrown into the waste paper bin. Watson recounts fantastic theories, scribbling on old newspapers and at a later stage the building of all kinds of possible models of the molecule.

But these were also years of serious and hard work, with an endless devotion to unveil the mystery.

Until finally in 1953, the only possible solution for the structure of DNA emerged. We still had to wait until the eighties before this solution could actually be verified with advanced research equipment and confirmed with a photograph.

Many scientists think the discovery of the structure of DNA is one of the most important findings of the last century. Through the DNA molecule it is possible to investigate everything related to heredity.

In 1962, Watson and Crick together with their colleague Maurice Wilkins received the Nobel Prize for Physiology or Medicine for their discovery.

Reproduction

The existence of the DNA molecule had already been discovered at the end of the 19th century. In the first half of the 20th century, it became clear DNA contains genetic information and thus plays a part in heredity. But how the molecule is built was learned only much later. As of that moment, researchers could begin to unravel how DNA operates.

DNA is one of the four molecules of life, indispensable for the creation of life. DNA and its related nucleic acid RNA are responsible for reproduction.

The other molecules of life are proteins that help molecules bond with each other and thus form larger entities; carbohydrates that provide fuel support; and lipids, molecules that don't dissolve in water and serve as cell membranes to separate cells from their environment.

DNA consists of a string of basic building blocks called nucleotides. Every nucleotide contains three smaller molecules: a phosphate, a sugar, and a base.

Two strings of nucleotides together make up some kind of ladder. The phosphates and the sugars are the stiles of the ladder. The bases of the two opposite nucleotides bond together and form the steps of the ladder.

These base pairs contain the genetic code. The genetic code is all the information a cell needs to reproduce itself and run its chemical factories. Make the ladder twist continuously and you end up with the DNA molecule.

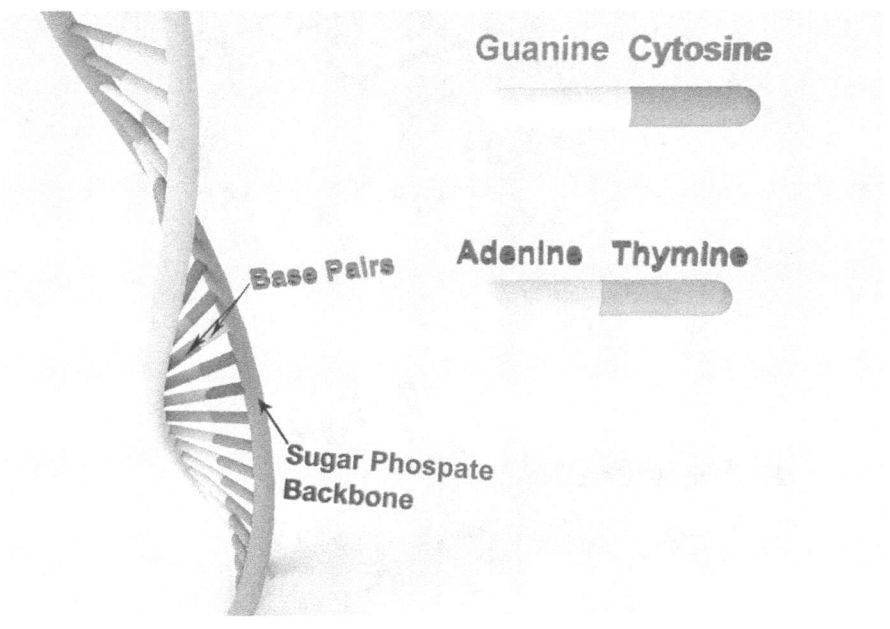

(© Giovanni Cancemi - fotolia.com)

The structure of DNA. The base pairs, forming the steps of the ladder, contain the genetic code.

Two

Every human cell holds 23 pairs of chromosomes. Half of them originate from your father, the other half comes from your mother. A chromosome is made up of one very long

DNA molecule. Different parts of DNA have different tasks, some of which are not known yet. The segments of DNA that contain hereditary information are called genes. Many genes can fit along the ladder of a single DNA molecule. The human genome comprises around 20.000 genes, according to the latest view among scientists worldwide.

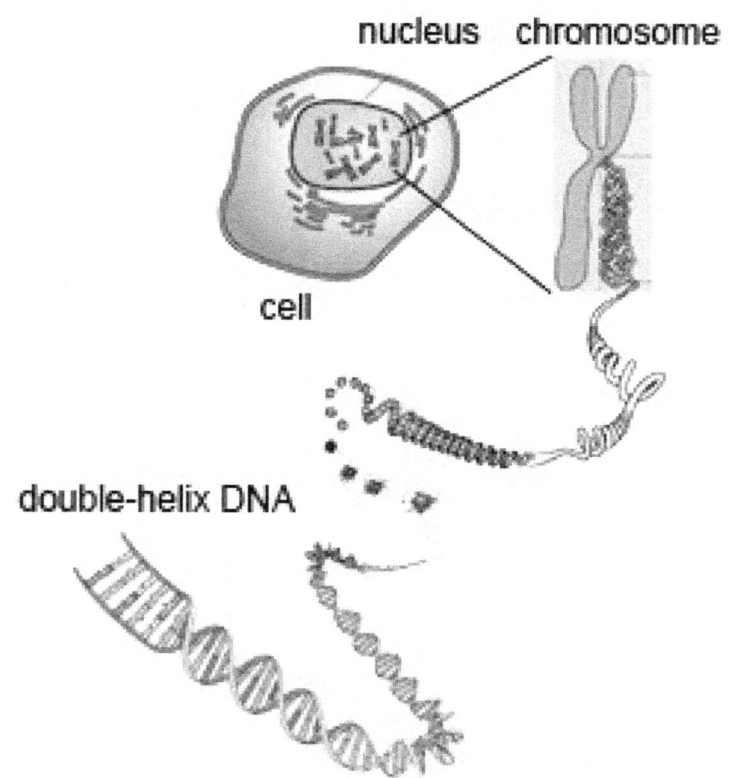

nucleus   chromosome

cell

double-helix DNA

(The brain from top to bottom)

Our cells carry a copy of two complete sets of the human genome spread out on 23 pairs of chromosomes in their nucleus. A chromosome is made up of one very long DNA molecule.

Different organisms have different numbers of genes. Mice and flies have more or less the same number of genes as humans; roundworms get along with around 13.000 genes. Certain crustaceans have over 30.000 genes and some plants more than 50.000. It is clear the number of genes is no measure for the state of development of an organism. What does count is how the organism uses its genes.

The cells in our body are small in size, but huge in complexity. It is very hard to imagine one cell contains not only several machineries to survive and function, but also our complete package of hereditary information.

Every cell in our body, except the red blood cells, carries in its nucleus a copy of two complete sets of the human genome – i.e. all 20.000 genes – spread out on 23 pairs of chromosomes. One set comes from your father and the other one from your mother.

Just think all this arises from that one sperm cell of father and that one egg cell of mother!

Book

The very special thing about the genome is it can copy itself to create a new cell, which again contains a complete genome. Genes hold the information necessary to build and maintain cells. Depending on the place in the body where the cell finds itself, different genes from the genome are active.

Whenever a gene is operational it results in the production of proteins. Almost everything in our body is made out of or by proteins, from every hair on our head to the hormones that make us interested in sex.

Genes also pass on hereditary traits to offspring this way. Some of these traits immediately catch the eye, like hair colour or the number of legs of an animal. Other traits are invisible, like musical talent or the risk to suffer certain diseases.

You can compare our genome with a book. Everybody has its own, unique book of life. Half of the chapters in that book have been derived from your father's book, the other half from your mother's book. During your growth in your mother's womb your book is being read and you come into being this way: with the blue eyes of your father and the blond hair of your mother for example.

No book is perfect. All books of life contain typographical errors. This can cause something to go wrong while your book is being read. These errors in the genome are responsible for instance for the birth of a child with Down syndrome, or spina bifida, or cleft lip.

At the moment of your birth, the book has not nearly been finished. It continues to be read during your whole life. Which chapter is being read depends on what you are doing, with what kind of substances you come into contact, what kind of food you take in. To formulate it more biologically correct: genes are being switched on and off.

Although our genetic code determines for an important part who and what we are, a strong connection also exists between genes and their environment.

A lot of attention has been given to heredity and destiny written in one's genes since the mapping of the human genome at the beginning of the 21st century. But genes need to be switched on or off to start chain reactions, which may lead to diseases. External events and free-willed behaviour are causing this switching off or on of genes.

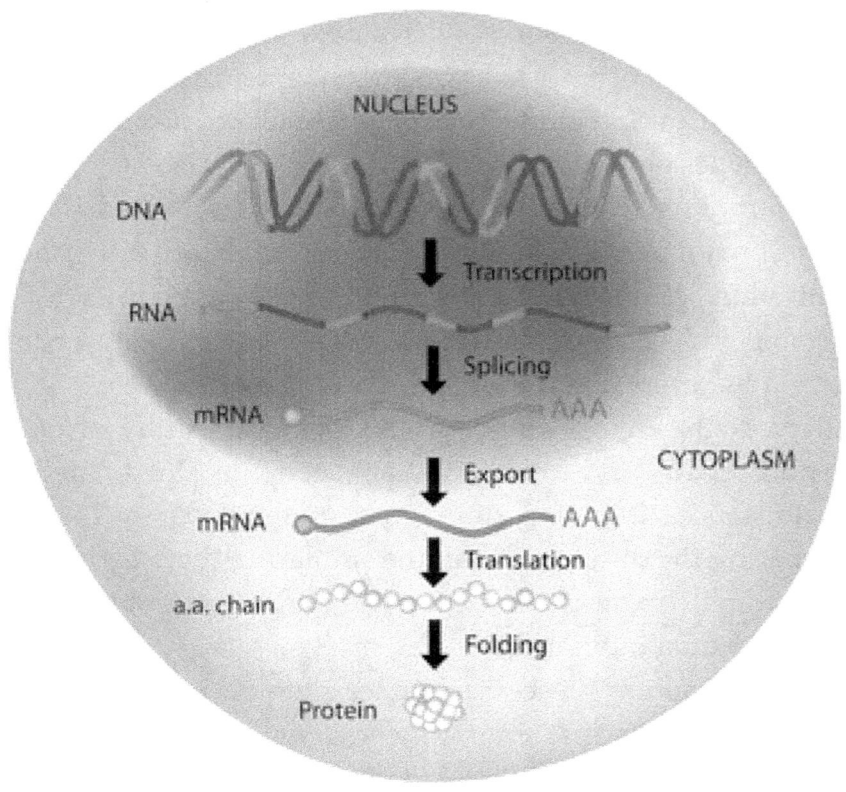

The segments of DNA that contain hereditary information are called genes. Genes hold the information necessary to build and maintain cells. Whenever a gene is activated it results in the production of proteins. Almost everything in our body is made out of or by proteins.

Specific molecules in the body send signals to genes to become operational or to shut down, in other words they switch genes on or off. This is a dynamical process that is strongly influenced by the environment. What someone eats; in what environment someone lives; exercise; stress; the drugs someone takes; or toxic substances that enter the body; all these factors influence the functioning of the molecules that switch genes on or off.

For example, scientists in the United States discovered air pollution not only is bad for your lungs and heart, but also for your brain. Long-lasting exposure to smog apparently affects learning and memory and aggravates anxiety and depression. To find out more about the influence of genes and what difference the environment makes, researchers study twins. Identical twins have exactly the same genome. Due to life's circumstances, they sometimes grow up far apart. By comparing the differences and the similarities between each half of the twin, much can be learned about genetic and environmental influences.

A word of caution is necessary concerning the outcomes of these studies. The first environment which exerts its influence is of course the mother's womb in which the embryo is developing. This explains for instance the extremely damaging impact of alcohol and nicotine on the unborn baby. Naturally, for both halves of the twin, although growing up apart, the womb environment had been the same.

Invisible

This means it certainly is not true that you find yourself at the mercy of the genes with which you were born. Naturally you cannot change the colour of your eyes. You will have to be satisfied with certain physical properties with which you came into this world, although some parts of your appearance could possibly be modified via plastic surgery. But, invisibly to you, your genome includes defective genes as well. And those defects may make you susceptible for instance to obesity or contribute to the development of a particular disease.

The emphasis in this matter is on the word 'may'. Because even though your genome contains a gene with a particular defect, it isn't necessarily the case this defective gene will actually be switched on. As long as the defective gene isn't activated the chain reaction causing the damage in your body isn't going to start. By sticking to a healthy lifestyle you can exert a lot of influence on whether or not genes will be activated.

Instead of us finding ourselves at the mercy of our genes you could even declare our genes depend on us, on how we choose to live. If you go bungee jumping for example stress will rush through your body. A large amount of the stress hormone cortisol will become available. This cortisol will go ranting back and forth switching on genes. It prepares your body for fight or flight. In prehistoric times, this was the first built-in reaction to dangerous, stressful situations.

The brain as it is now, originated about one hundred thousand years ago, when homo sapiens, modern man, started to populate earth.

That is why we often still can react so primitively. We acquired our brain in the ages of the cave-dwellers. It hasn't been designed for driving a car, traveling in an airplane, using mobile telephones and computers.

Therefore, our brain still prepares our body for fight or flight in stressful situations, although nowadays fight and flight are on the bottom of the list of possible reactions to a problematic situation. Even in dangerous situations you opted for yourself, like in the case of bungee jumping, the preparation for fight or flight is started automatically. That is why stress can be so damaging in the long run. The genes activated by the cortisol, may be involved in the development of diseases.

Complicated

Where you are and what you are doing thus determines which chapters in your book of life, your genome, will be opened. If a chapter with an erroneous text is being read, something goes wrong and this could start a process which ends with you getting a disease. By the way, there are only very few diseases that arise because of a defect in just one gene. Generally, various genes with defects have to be switched on to give rise to a disease.

In the whole world, scientists are busy finding out which defective genes are involved in which diseases. In most cases, it is terribly difficult to discover a direct link between specific genes and particular biological processes or diseases. Often complicated mechanisms are going on, in which different genes play a role.

This observation led to huge disappointment after about ten years have passed since the mapping of the human genome. Ten years ago, great enthusiasm had taken the scientific community. Expectations were very high. It was thought the functions of the different genes could be determined rapidly. This was supposed to lead quickly to the development of drugs for the diseases caused by these genes. The whole system results to be far more complicated than anticipated at first and progress is exasperatingly slow.

But progress there is, even though the steps forward are small and not always earth-shattering.

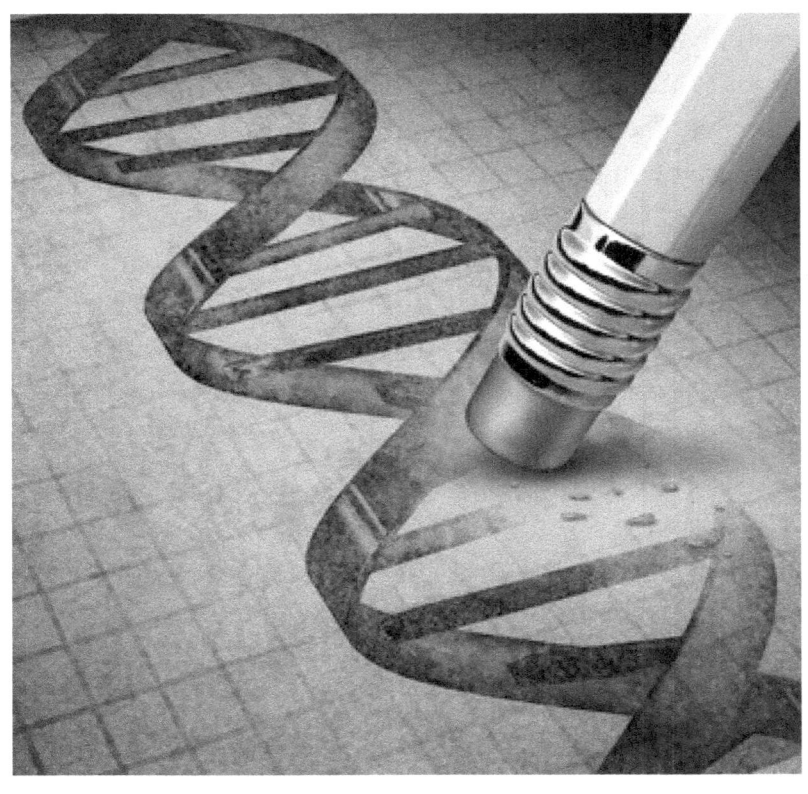

Manipulating defective genes is only possible via highly elaborate gene therapies.

One of the main conclusions so far is that for the time being attention particularly has to be given to a healthy lifestyle. As stated earlier, a healthy lifestyle has a very positive influence on whether or not genes will be switched on. Manipulating defective genes is only possible via highly elaborate gene therapies. Defective genes could perhaps be repaired this way or they could be replaced by new, healthy genes.
In laboratory animals, genetic manipulation is employed

extensively already, but for human beings no successful treatments are available yet. Actually, we don't fully know thus far what will be the consequences of what we are doing where genetic manipulation is concerned. Interfering in such a complex process brings about huge risks.

For example, via an experimental gene therapy treatment in a group of persons, the deadly disease concerned admittedly was brought under control, but at the same time genes involved in cancer were activated due to which some of the participants developed leukaemia.

Prevent

So, it is important not to rely too much upon the fact that soon methods will become available to tinker with your genes. As far as genes are concerned for the time being, preventing is the only option since curing is no alternative yet.

That being so, it is wise to take matters in your own hands and make sure your gene collection stays as healthy as possible. Therefore, you have to try to live in a way that will skip certain unhealthy chapters in your book of life.

Sometimes, it may be useful to know which chapters in your personal book of life contain errors. If for instance a hereditary disease runs in your family and it is known which defects in which genes would contribute to the development of the disease, you might want to know whether you carry those defective genes.

A very clear case of such a hereditary disease is Huntington's disease, an incurable disorder that damages parts of the brain, affects muscle coordination and leads to cognitive decline. Huntington's disease is hereditary and is caused by just one defective gene. When father or mother carries this faulty gene children have a fifty percent chance to also get the disease. But carriers of the Huntington's gene often don't know their genome contains this defect before they already have had children. The disease manifests itself only in adult life, mostly between 35 and 45 years of age.

In such a case it is fantastic of course that nowadays the possibility exists to perform a genetic test to check if someone carries the Huntington's gene. However, some people don't want to know whether or not they carry defective genes involved in a serious disease. They prefer to wait and see. This is a choice everybody has to make on their own.

In the case of Huntington's disease, it turns out only five percent of people at risk want to undergo genetic screening. Knowing that in about twenty years' time you will succumb to a disease with a terrible degenerating course, while you are still in perfect health at the moment, is a burden almost impossible to bear. Persons in that situation often choose a fairly normal life in the healthy years ahead, although in the background the dark threat of the disease constantly looms.

Testing

Genetic testing is becoming ever more popular. A series of different genetic tests exist. The best-known is the DNA test that can determine if two people are related to one another. This is used for instance when someone is trying to find his or her biological father or mother. DNA tests are also employed in court, for example to find out whether the semen found came from the suspect in a sex crime.

In this type of genetic tests, laboratory assistants only study the DNA molecule as it has been taken from a person concerned and compare this with the other DNA molecule involved. Other kinds of genetic screening are about finding genetic defects. These are about the search for abnormalities in chromosomes, genes, or proteins.

A question that needs to be answered is what use the results of such tests may have. Companies that look to hire someone may stop the procedure when a genetic test of the candidate has shown certain defects. Insurance companies may refuse to cover a potential customer carrying some defective genes that appear to be involved in the development of cancer. And you yourself may forget to enjoy life if you are afraid to get certain diseases that are connected to some abnormalities in your genome.

The consequences of having this information could potentially be rather dramatic. This is even more of a shame since hardly any clarity exists, apart from a few exceptions, which defects in which genes could eventually be the cause of which diseases. Besides, the genes concerned should have to be switched on to actually start the disease process. And this switching on of genes is partially your own doing.

Researchers of the University of Goteborg in Sweden came up with solid proof for this. They investigated the connection between the genes you were born with and the age you would reach at your death.

Their conclusion is that the age your parents reached isn't of great influence. It certainly is not a fact that you will become about just as old as your parents because of the genes you inherited from them.

Of far more importance is how and where you live. According to the study, your life expectancy is determined for more than 75 percent by the environment in which you live and by your lifestyle.

Genes are important. They hold the directions for the initial growth of the brain. But they don't have the final say since they don't control how the brain will react. Everything we do influences every process that follows in the brain. From conception to death, our genes and the environment interact and constantly change our brain.

6. ETERNAL YOUTH

What is ageing?

We all age. As a child, we love to age and can't wait to finally become an adult. But when you are in your thirties, already growing older is associated with negative feelings: decline, diseases, loneliness, death. They are phantoms we prefer to put away in dark closets. Often, we try to counteract the signs of ageing with all kinds of artificial interventions. It isn't enough anymore to simply dye your grey hairs. Complete bodies have to be renovated. The most outrageous and above all expensive therapies go like hot cakes, especially among people who have built their entire existence upon their beautiful looks. But in the end, there is no escape. We will age. The years just accumulate. This is a process of physical, psychological and social changes.

The life expectancy of man has risen quite a bit in the past decennia. For thousands of years, our average life expectancy was about forty years. Thanks to better nourishment and advanced medical care, people nowadays live considerably longer. In most developed countries, life expectancy has reached eighty years at the moment and the rise hasn't come to a stop yet. But there are also exceptions. In the southern part of Africa for instance, life expectancy has decreased due to the rise of AIDS. And also in Russia, life has become less healthy after the fall of the Soviet Union. For men, life expectancy at the moment does not reach sixty years of age there. The United States and Japan on the contrary, count the largest numbers of centenarians among their inhabitants. Researchers expect half of the baby's born there since the year 2000 to reach the age of ninety and ten percent will get to one hundred.

The situation is different when you talk about life span. Every organism has a maximum life span. This maximum is more or less fixed. For human beings, the maximum life span is around 125 years of age. But we are well overtaken by the Galapagos tortoise that can reach 190 years of age, a type of shark and a type of whale that can become 200 years of age, and a type of Japanese fish that amply surpasses those 200 years. A bivalve mollusc tops the list with a maximum life span of 405 to 410 years. How do we know that? By counting the yearly growth lines on their valves, just like in trees. Mice on the other end of the spectrum only reach the age of four, dogs will not live into their thirties, and cats aren't going to pass the age of forty. Trees seem to be able to grow for thousands of years and nobody knows whether they then die because of old age. One organism certainly is not dying of old age: the jellyfish turritopsis nutricula. After this jellyfish has reached maturity and has procreated, it returns to its youthful form. This cycle can go on endlessly. Theoretically this makes this jellyfish immortal, unless it succumbs to a disease or is eaten by a predator, which is almost always the case.

Process
What does it mean, ageing, in the biological sense and why does the maximum life span differ so much for various life forms? The jury is still out on this one. Ageing is about biological changes that gradually take place within an organism after reaching sexual maturity. In the end, ageing

leads to the death of an organism although ageing is not a cause of death. For death to occur, always a more direct cause exists, in the form of some disease.

In general, genetic as well as environmental factors contribute to the ageing process. People, who live under extreme circumstances, grow old sooner. This has to do with among other things the fact that their cells suffer a lot.

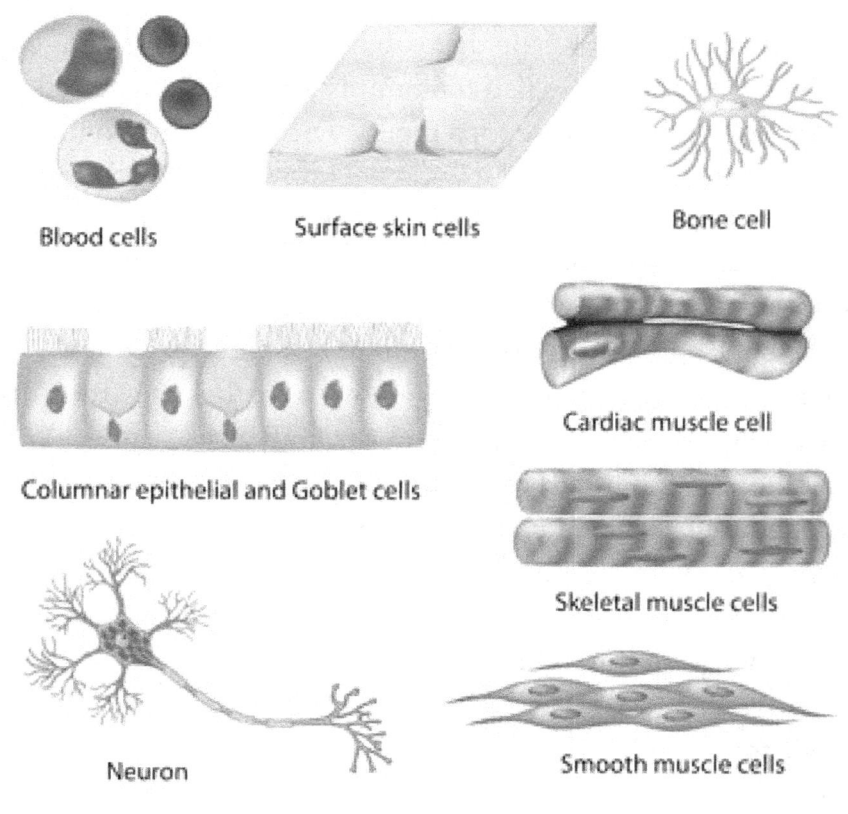

Blood cells

Surface skin cells

Bone cell

Columnar epithelial and Goblet cells

Cardiac muscle cell

Skeletal muscle cells

Neuron

Smooth muscle cells

(© Alila Medical Media - Fotolia.com)

Human cell collection. Environmental factors influence the health of cells and thus contribute to the ageing process.

One of the theories on ageing is about free radicals. Radicals are unstable oxygen molecules that take part in important biological processes. They come into being during normal metabolism in cells.

Radicals contain an unpaired electron, which reacts with electrons from neighbouring molecules. This is called oxidation and damages the molecule involved. Free radicals can thus damage DNA, proteins, and cell membranes. An excess of radicals may be caused by eating in a bad way. If you eat a lot of fried food for instance many saturated fats enter the body and these are a source for the formation of free radicals.

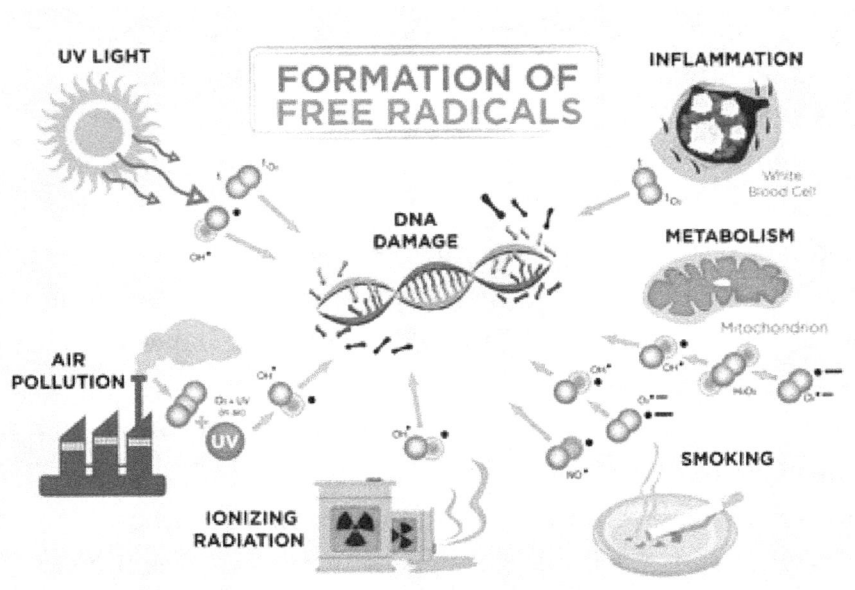

(© crystaleyestudio)

Fortunately, our bodies possess a safety system in the form of antioxidants. In normal situations, these antioxidants are capable of stabilising the radicals and thus render them harmless. Sometimes the safety system fails and it cannot prevent damage caused by radicals from happening. Radicals are involved in a very extensive range of diseases, among which Parkinson disease, schizophrenia, bipolar disorder, cardiovascular disease, chronic fatigue syndrome, and Alzheimer disease. And they probably also play a part in the ageing process, when the antioxidants' line of defence is no longer a match for the continuous stream of radicals.

Superfluous

Specialists in evolution theory come up with a more general explanation for the ageing process. According to them, the speed with which different organisms grow older has to do with their genetic make-up. Every organism may have been fitted with a kind of survival program that functions well until the moment an individual becomes superfluous. That moment of superfluity is mainly defined by the maximum age at which an organism is still able to procreate. To state it more clearly: the various body parts will last just long enough to see its children mature.

Genes involved in damage to the body before or during the time of reproduction will automatically become extinct through natural selection. Individuals, who carry these damaging genes, will die young and won't have the time to reproduce. Thus they won't pass on the genes concerned to their offspring. Individuals, who do not carry the damaging genes, do procreate. In the course of time, no carriers of the damaging genes will be left.

The situation is very different for the time after the period of reproduction. Genes that could set in motion a chain of decline and disease won't be eliminated by natural selection. The carriers of these damaging genes have reproduced already and will have passed on the genes to their offspring. It is also possible these genes that are damaging at a later age may have had useful tasks earlier in life. This could be an explanation for the fact that diseases continue to exist in the course of evolution. According to this theory, ageing is not an inevitable quality of living, but the result of genetic programming.

Copies

Various hundreds of genes have already been pinpointed as being involved in the ageing process, but how this involvement goes about is still unclear. Ageing actually is a simultaneous deterioration of various body systems. Genes that play a part in the functioning of each of these systems, carry part of the responsibility for the ageing process. Something that really is of great importance is the maximum number of times a cell can split itself to form two new copies. Cells are constantly being copied. This process starts with that one fused egg and sperm cell containing 46 chromosomes, 23 of father and 23 of mother, with the complete genome. Every chromosome in fact is a very long DNA molecule holding several hundreds of genes. While copying this large package of information something can easily go wrong. Especially when you consider the fact that one copy follows another and another to finally end up with a complete human being. And this copying process of cells continues throughout your whole life.

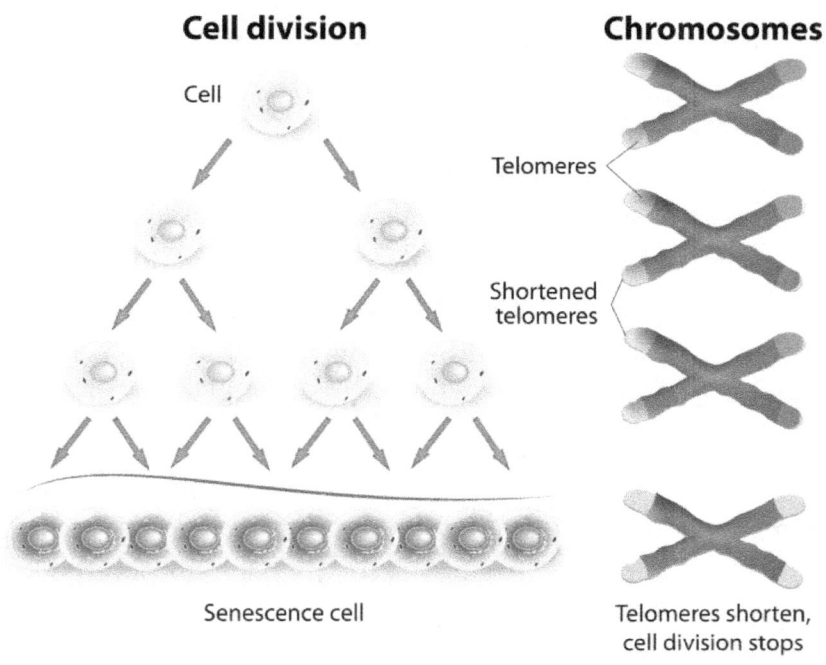

Cell division

Cell

Senescence cell

Chromosomes

Telomeres

Shortened telomeres

Telomeres shorten, cell division stops

(© designua - Fotolia.com)

The copying process of cells continues throughout life. Every time a cell is copied a small part of telomere, an irrelevant part, disappears. When all the telomere is gone the cell cannot copy anymore. This generally leads to the death of the cell.

Copies aren't always as good as the original. To prevent damage due to the copying process every DNA molecule is fitted with an irrelevant, extra part at the beginning and the end of the molecule, called telomere. Compare the situation to a photocopier that can't copy a complete page. The upper and lower edges of the paper are not completely clear anymore. To prevent important text to be left out, all the pages to be copied start and end with some nonsense lines. This way, the indispensable information will certainly be on your copy. But every time you make a new copy of the copy, again a part of the nonsense lines at the top and the bottom of the page will disappear. You will end up with a copy that does not contain nonsense lines anymore, but only the relevant information. You cannot afford to lose this important information, so you have to stop copying.

This is what happens in cell division. With every new copy a small piece of telomere is left off. When all the telomere has gone, the cell cannot divide anymore. This almost always leads to the death of the cell. So, the shrinking telomere makes cells grow older.

In the brain, neurones do not duplicate, but glial cells do and thus suffer from too much copying.

It appears the length of the telomere determines the maximum life span of an organism. In humans, telomeres have such a length they can easily survive 75 to 90 years. Human cells can divide between forty and sixty times before they have run out of telomere. Cells of mice can be copied about fifteen times, but the cells of the Galapagos tortoise at least ninety times.

Length

The length of the telomeres appears to vary a little between persons. If your parents had long telomeres you will inherit long telomeres as well. But it certainly does not mean this fact guarantees that you will reach about the same age as your parents did, as was shown in the above mentioned Swedish investigation. Environmental factors have a far bigger influence on telomere length. When cells are damaged faster than usual and have to be replaced, more cell divisions take place in a shorter period and telomere runs out quicker. For example, stress or a large quantity of free radicals influences telomere length.

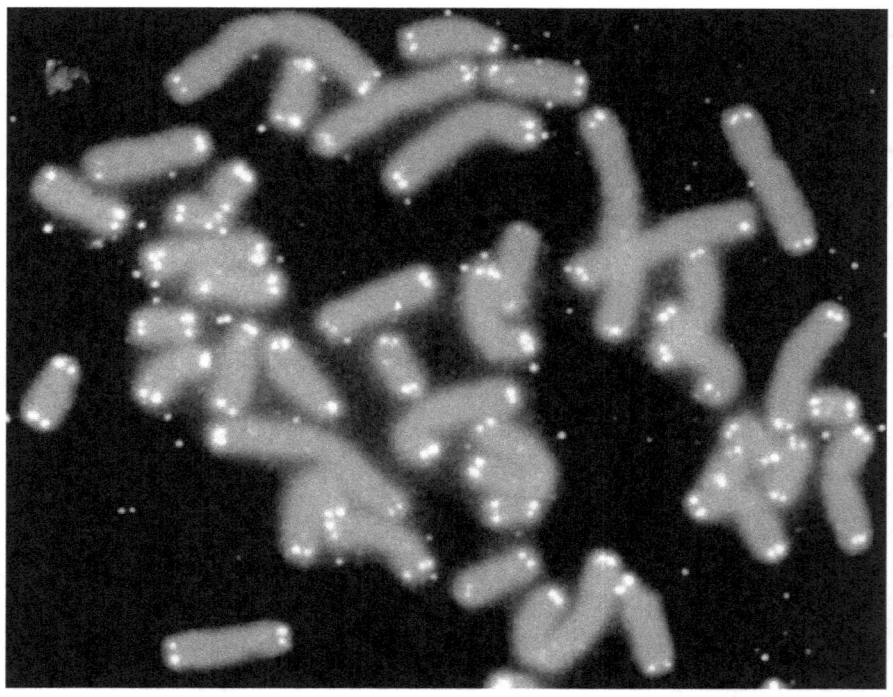

© U.S. Department of Energy Human Genome Program

Human chromosomes capped by telomeres.

Telomere length is an interesting measure for how far the ageing process has affected your body. With this measure, researchers in the US have been able to establish that chronic stress makes you grow older faster. They investigated two groups of mothers. One group had healthy children while the other group was taking care of chronically ill children what caused these women to be exposed to long-term stress.

In the stressed mothers the telomeres turned out to be considerably shorter than in the mothers with healthy children. Depending on the period they had already been taking care of their chronically ill child, they appeared between nine and seventeen years older as far as telomere length was concerned.

Telomere length may also have to do with the premature death of the famous Dolly, a cloned sheep. Cloning is an artificial reproduction method meant to create identical offspring, a clone.

Dolly was the first cloned mammal. She was born in 1996 in Scotland. To create her, DNA material of one sheep was inserted into an egg cell from which the nucleus was removed, of another sheep. The fertilised egg was placed into the womb of a third sheep and she gave birth to Dolly.

Genetically speaking, Dolly had only one parent. She was an identical descendant of the sheep of which the DNA had been taken.

Dolly died in 2003 at the age of six. Normally, sheep of the species Dolly belonged to will live to be eleven or twelve years old.

An investigation after Dolly's death revealed her telomeres were far shorter than those of other sheep of six years old. This may have been caused by the fact that when the cloning took place the telomeres involved were shorter than normal even then. The sheep of which the DNA had been used was six years of age and its telomeres already had been shortened because of previous cell divisions.

Dolly's creator, Ian Wilmut, contradicts this explanation and maintains Dolly died of a lung disease which is very common in sheep. Of course it could also be that the sheep succumbed to the lung disease, because her cells had aged already and couldn't handle the disease anymore.

Rejuvenation

Telomeres don't always only become shorter. A special protein, telomerase, is able to repair both ends of the DNA molecule and lengthens the telomere up to its original length. Telomerase is made by one of our genes and could give a cell eternal life.

Unfortunately, this gene is active for only a short period of time, mainly in egg cells and sperm cells. After all, they are the originals for all the copies that will follow. In an embryo that develops normally, the genes that make telomerase are switched off.

Even in adults, telomerase can still be found, namely in cells of the immune system. These have to keep on dividing themselves to effectively protect the body against intruders, like viruses, bacteria and parasites.

Cancer cells also make use of, or in fact abuse, telomerase. They are capable of switching on the gene that produces telomerase. Thanks to this ability they can duplicate infinitely. One of the paths being followed in cancer research at the moment is aimed at this activation of the telomerase gene by cancer cells. The search is on for a method to counteract the production of telomerase triggered by cancer cells. If that would be possible cancer cells would automatically die because they would run out of telomere due to their frequent cell division.

TELOMERASE

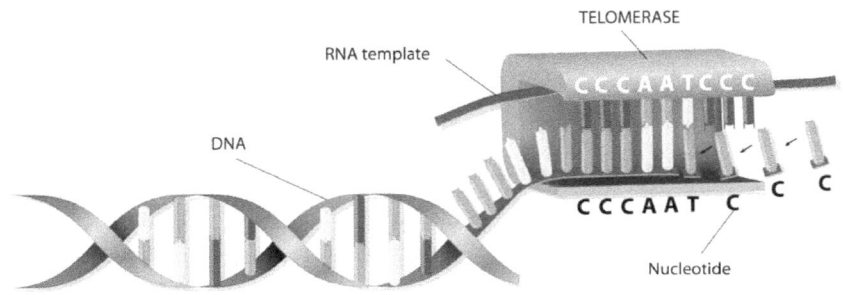

(© designua - Fotolia.com)

A special protein called telomerase is able to lengthen telomeres again. The genes that make telomerase are shut off when an embryo is developing normally. Cancer cells are able to switch these genes on again and can thus duplicate infinitely.

After the discovery of telomeres and telomerase, naturally scientists thought they had found the fountain of youth. If we could activate telomerase genes and thus lengthen our telomeres time and again our cells would become immortal. In the laboratory, cells that had been genetically manipulated and that kept on producing telomerase, in fact were able to divide unlimited.

Tests have also been done in genetically modified mice. From the moment the telomerase gene was switched on in the mice, they underwent a complete rejuvenation. Most of those mice on the other hand fell ill with cancer and still died prematurely. Cancer cells use the telomerase gene as well, as explained earlier. Only mice that had been made cancer proof via another genetic intervention indeed lived longer.

The question is how far you could go intervening in genetic processes without upsetting the whole complicated and ingenious process.

A telomerase therapy for humans still seems to be a long way off. For the time being, we will have to deal with our ageing cells and try to find ways to keep them healthy as long as possible.

7. STANDING STRONG TOGETHER

The resilience of our brain

Our brain is amazingly adept in standing up to the ravages of time. Until very recently, it was thought growing old brought along only distress and misery. After a spike between our thirties and our fifties, the brain's functioning would only deteriorate. Brain cells would go under by the hundreds and this would result in a continuous decline of our cognitive abilities.

In practice, this worst-case scenario frequently doesn't become a reality. Many famous people delivered their best performances at advanced age.

Grandma Moses of the US for instance started painting when she was 76 years old. During the fifties, when she already was in her nineties, her exhibitions drew large crowds worldwide. Pianist Arthur Rubinstein of Polish origin gave one of his best concerts in New York when he had already turned 89. Writer Harry Bernstein, a Brit emigrated to the US, published his debut novel at age 96. The American astronaut John Glenn at 77 years of age became the oldest person ever in space on board of the Space Shuttle Discovery.

These famous people aren't the only ones that lead an interesting and pleasant life at advanced age. We all know people in our vicinity that may be old in years, but not in how they live and how they behave themselves. They are vivacious people, wise and sharp, full of wit and of whom you think: that's the way I would like to grow old. On the other hand, everybody also knows elderly in their surroundings who suffer dementia and from whom their spirit is slowly slipping away.

What is happening in our brain during the ageing process what makes these differences arise?

Unique

The human brain goes through quite a number of changes before a child is born. At the moment of birth, the brain structure is more or less ready, but for many years work is still going on filling in details. During all of our lives, new connections are made between brain cells while other connections are broken. This process is influenced by what we do and how and where we live.

So, although all brains have the same general features, neural connections are distinctive. This makes every brain unique, formed by individual experiences.

What happens to the brain past the reproductive age is still open to discussion. It was thought that the death of cells caused significant brain atrophy. The folds of the cortex seemed to be flattening and the cortex itself appeared to become thinner.

Research even seemed to reveal these changes were more intense in men than in women. New imaging techniques available nowadays have made it possible to investigate the brain in very fine detail.

These new investigations brought out other results. Earlier study results may also have become clouded due to the participation of older adults without symptoms of dementia and thus without the diagnosis, but with initial dementia processes going on in their brains. Now, when elderly people are being asked to participate in a research project, first their brains are mapped completely with scanners to see whether some kind of disease process is already going on that would make the results of the research project invalid.

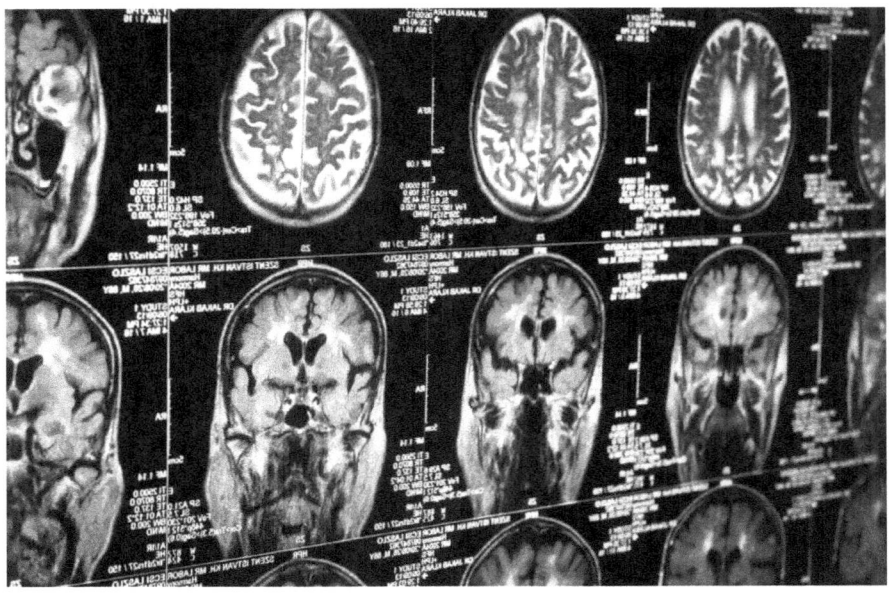

(© svedoliver - Fotolia.com)

Thanks to imaging techniques that result in sharp scans, it is possible to investigate the brain in very fine detail.

According to the latest state of affairs, normal ageing of the brain is not accompanied by the death of large quantities of brain cells. Our brains do not shrink notably. Nor do clear differences exist between the ageing of the male and the female brain. Extensive differences however do exist between the ageing processes in individual brains.

Less

In general, while ageing, the brain weight may decrease. This is caused by the fact that in certain parts of the brain somewhat more neurones die.

The hippocampus, which we already encountered in chapter 2, is such a vulnerable area. This tiny structure in the centre of the brain is very vulnerable to long-term stress. Because the hippocampus plays a very important part in our memory, loss of neurones in that area may be the cause of memory problems at advanced age.

In some elderly, movements get slower and less fluent. This might be due to the fact that neurones die in another sensitive brain area, the substantia nigra. This structure is a decisive factor in the development of Parkinson disease, a disease that is accompanied by severe disturbances in locomotion.

Where brain areas shrink the open space is taken over by the ventricle system, four interconnected cavities filled with cerebrospinal fluid. These cavities slowly enlarge with age.

Information transfer between neurones could also become a bit more difficult at advanced age. This is caused by the fact that lesser quantities of neurotransmitters are available. These neurotransmitters are necessary to transfer information from one neurone to the next.

Besides, in the course of time some plaques, clots of waste from brain metabolism, may appear in the space between brain cells. These plaques hamper a smooth flow of information.

A reduced cerebral blood flow is also part of the normal ageing process. Blood vessels become less supple while ageing. This results in less oxygen brought to the brain. A shortage of oxygen may lead to the death of neurones.

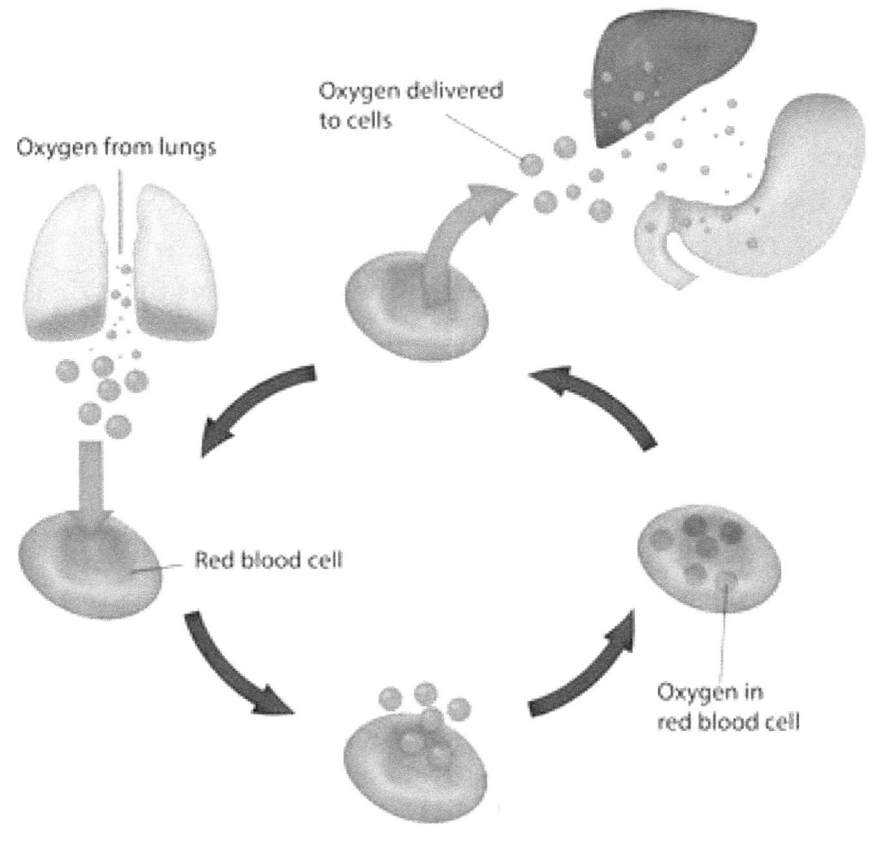

Oxygen delivered to cells

Oxygen from lungs

Red blood cell

Oxygen in red blood cell

(© joshya - Fotolia.com)

Red blood cells bring oxygen from the lungs to cells throughout the body. As part of the ageing process, less blood flows to the brain. The brain receives less oxygen which may lead to the death of neurones.

An interesting development during the ageing process is that both hemispheres lose a little of their specialisation. Over the years, they cooperate more closely. Activities that used to take place in one hemisphere increasingly occupy both hemispheres. It seems this way the brain finds a solution for a less effective single hemisphere. The hemispheres stand stronger together.

Plasticity

On the neuronal level, the ageing brain unifies forces as well. Where neurones drop out and die, neighbouring neurones help out to keep networks going. The brain seems to rewire. Responsibilities for a given task can be shifted from one region to another.

This is a phenomenon that goes on throughout your life. It is called neuroplasticity. Everything we do, learn, and think influences the structure and organisation of the brain. This is possible thanks to the fact that neurones can adapt their activity in reaction to changes in their environment. Besides, they can fulfil more than one function simultaneously.

For example, when you learn another language the brain parts involved in language are being used intensively. These parts become larger because neighbouring neurones are called upon for assistance to get the extra work done.

The most obvious example for plasticity in the human brain is the brain of a blind person.

The brain part that is normally used for the processing of information entering via the eyes is taken over in blind people by the part that processes tactile information. This way, a larger brain area is available for the information coming from the finger tips which is very important due to the absence of visual input.

Studies involving persons who had just gone blind and volunteers wearing a blindfold showed that this type of reorganisation within the brain can happen in a matter of days. In a similar way, in deaf people the brain's visual part annexes the neuronal networks that normally would process information coming from the ears.

A very special case of neuroplasticity takes place in people who have lost a leg, an arm, or a hand. In about 95 percent of amputees, a syndrome occurs called phantom limb syndrome. They have feelings of sensation in the missing limb. The phantom limb syndrome often persists for a lifetime.

The cause of this syndrome can probably be found in the workings of neuroplasticity. The neural networks that were connected to the limb that now isn't there anymore are still intact. Nearby neural networks are trying to recruit the inactive neurones.

Thus neural networks reorganise themselves to take over an area of the brain that the body is no longer using. Touch receptors in the body part that is taking over, form connections with neurones in the cortex that were normally contacted by receptors in the missing limb. When the body part that has innervated the free space is stimulated, higher brain areas continue to interpret the signals as arising from a limb that is no longer there.

Alternative

Phantom limb syndrome is an example of maladaptive plasticity. But in evolution, the benefits of a plastic brain that can adapt to a changing environment far outweigh this disadvantage.

Neuroplasticity is greatest during development of the brain. In early childhood, when a part of the brain is damaged, the function that used to be performed by this part may shift to another area. After some time, the child performs the same as other children.

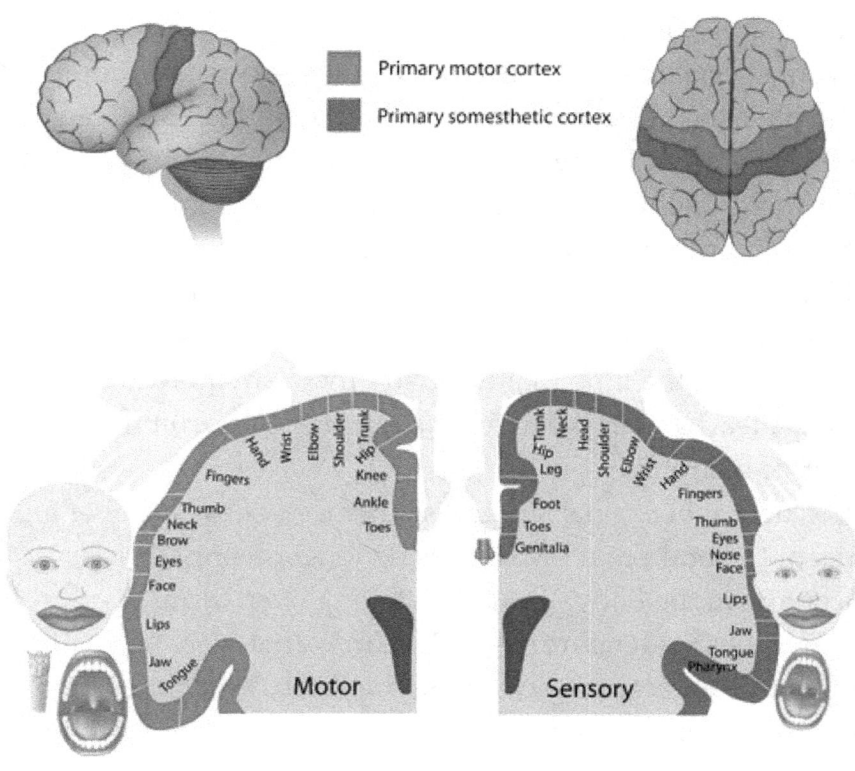

Primary motor cortex

Primary somesthetic cortex

Motor

Sensory

(© Alila Medical Media)

*Special parts of the brain are dedicated to movement and other parts
to the senses. Within these parts, every body part has its own
segment. These networks are not fixed. They get bigger or smaller
with the use we make of the body part concerned. This is called
neuroplasticity and goes on throughout our lives.*

Although the adult brain is relatively rigid, plasticity does
exist there also. Unemployed neurones are taken in by
neighbouring networks and waste areas get dedicated to
other tasks. In addition, the adult brain has the possibility to

100

figure out an alternative strategy to transfer information when the original route is blocked.

That's why it is useful and even necessary to continue learning throughout your life and undertake new activities at a regular basis. This creates new connections between brain cells. The more connections you have, the better it is. When you lose some connections from time to time due to for instance disease, a concussion, or toxic chemical substances you will have sufficient connections left. Detours will arise and the brain will still be able to perform as many of its functions as possible.

Reorganisation

Plasticity decreases with age, but the brain retains the ability to rewire itself throughout life. The adult brain not only forms new connections in response to changing environmental conditions, but can also rewire itself after some types of damage.

One of the first persons to discover this was the American brain scientist Paul Bach-y-Rita. His father had suffered a stroke. Despite extensive damage in his brain, with intensive training he succeeded to live a relatively normal life. After his death, autopsy revealed other parts of his brain had taken over the functions of the lost parts.

Bach-y-Rita dedicated the rest of his life to studying neuroplasticity. He has invented some ingenious machines that encourage damaged brains to reorganise.

An example is a brain machine for people with damage to their vestibular apparatus. Due to this damage the patient continuously loses his balance and falls frequently. The device consists of some accelerometers positioned on the body of the patient. Via a computer they send information on the body's position to a small plate on the patient's tongue. According to the position of the body different areas of the tongue are being stimulated. Thus the sensory receptors of the tongue take over the task of the vestibular apparatus.

In the end, the brain learns to translate signals that enter via the tongue, for the use of balancing the body. Over time, balance signals are sent automatically from the tongue to the brain forming new pathways. The patient then doesn't need the device anymore and is again able to keep his balance without a problem.

The brain's ability to reorganise is also used in a special rehabilitation program for people who have had a stroke and as a result ended up with a paralysed hand or arm. This paralysis occurs because a small part of the brain responsible for movement has been damaged during the stroke. The neurones in this area are dead or seriously injured. And this damage will spread because the patient is not using the paralysed limb. Neurones that don't receive signals anymore, because the neighbours are dead, will die as well.

Constraint-induced movement therapy forces the patient to use the affected limb by restricting the unaffected one. This stimulates the growth of new neural pathways.

The training uses skills closely related to everyday life. It is done in increments and concentrated into a short period. At a certain stage of the therapy, patients go out for a meal in a restaurant with their functioning arm or hand disabled in a sling. The staff has been informed of their visit beforehand since eating with hands or arms that don't function properly, logically results in quite a mess. The other guests look on open-mouthed.

But it does work! Thanks to a very intensive training and tons of perseverance, new connections are made in the damaged brain part that make the use of hand or arm possible again. Of course, this can only happen when after the stroke enough working neurones have been left in the vicinity to take over the job of the deceased neurones. In most cases, the reorganisation and rewiring aren't perfect, which makes the movements a bit clumsy, but the improvement is substantial in many cases.

It is a pity we are not so good at brain reorganisation as planarians, a flatworm type, one of the most primitive animals that have a brain. They have a very high regenerative capacity. If after amputation only a small piece of its body is left in which no brain tissue remains, a planarian can regenerate its entire body including its brain within five days.

Renew

Why is regeneration in humans so difficult then? From an evolutionary perspective, this might be linked to the fact that humans depend on what they've learned. An adult human cannot survive if after injury his brain is renewed and all previous knowledge is lost. Still, our brains are not only capable of reorganising, but are even able to renew themselves in the details. This process is called neurogenesis and comprises the birth of new neurones.

It has long been the general belief that new neurones only came into life during the development of the brain. At your birth, your brain came with an estimated one hundred billion neurones and that was all you were going to get to make it through your life. New neurones were not going to be added since neurones can't copy themselves like other cells can.

The fact that we cannot perceive something obviously doesn't mean it does not exist. In recent years, especially in brain research sure facts had to be revised. This was also the case with the birth of new neurones.

Recently, it has been shown without a shadow of a doubt that new neurones are also born into the adult brain, probably throughout its lifetime.

The first signs of neurones being born in an adult brain came from the brains of songbirds. The brains of male songbirds change with the mating season. They have to produce complex songs to attract females. When their blood levels of testosterone rise their vocal centres become bigger. New neurones formed in the ventricles migrate to the vocal centre. Thanks to this bigger vocal centre, the birds can sing impressively to conquer a female.

After years of disbelieving and having done away with evidence, brain scientists all over the world are finally convinced even in the adult human brain new neurones are being born.

With ageing, the birth of new neurones decreases, but neurogenesis is maintained at a very low level for most of the life span. Some scientists believe new neurones are born throughout the nervous system, but there's still no proof for that.

In several brain areas it is certain, though, new neurones are brought into action whenever necessary.

One of those areas is the hippocampus, already well-known to us. Since this part of the brain is essential for learning and memory, the new neurones are probably required for these tasks. If for some reason the production of new neurones ceases, problems arise. The hippocampus shrinks and it is getting harder to remember things, just like what happens in Alzheimer disease.

Stem cells

Neurones are not able to divide, as said before. But where do these new neurones come from then? This is where we touch the presently almost infamous stem cells. Stem cells are undifferentiated cells that have no identified or specialised function yet. They possess the ability to give rise to multiple distinct cell types. Stem cells eventually differentiate into cells of tissues and organs. An embryo starts out with only stem cells. As its development progresses, more and more of those stem cells are specialising and will get a specific function in the body.

Embryonic stem cells are very powerful. This is called pluripotent, which means they can generate all cell types in the body. That's why embryonic stem cells are so useful for stem cell therapies. Such therapies include implanting those stem cells into persons who suffer a certain disease. The idea is that the stem cells will replace ill or death cells. They could for instance form new skin cells in people with third degree burns or new bone marrow cells in people with leukaemia. Objections exist against the use of embryonic stem cells. Many people are opposed to the use of embryos on ethical grounds, mainly because of religious beliefs. They hold the view that an individual comes into being at the moment of conception and consider an embryo to be a human being. In addition, transplant of embryonic stem cells is not without danger for the receiver of the cells. They are foreign to the body and the patient needs special treatment because of rejection of the cells by the immune system.

That's why it was such a great discovery when it became clear adults also have stem cells in different tissues in their bodies. They have been found in for instance bone marrow, peripheral blood, dental pulp, skeletal muscle, skin tissue, liver, and pancreas.

In general, they generate cell types of the organ from which they originate to replenish dying cells and regenerate damaged tissue.

Human Stem Cell Applications

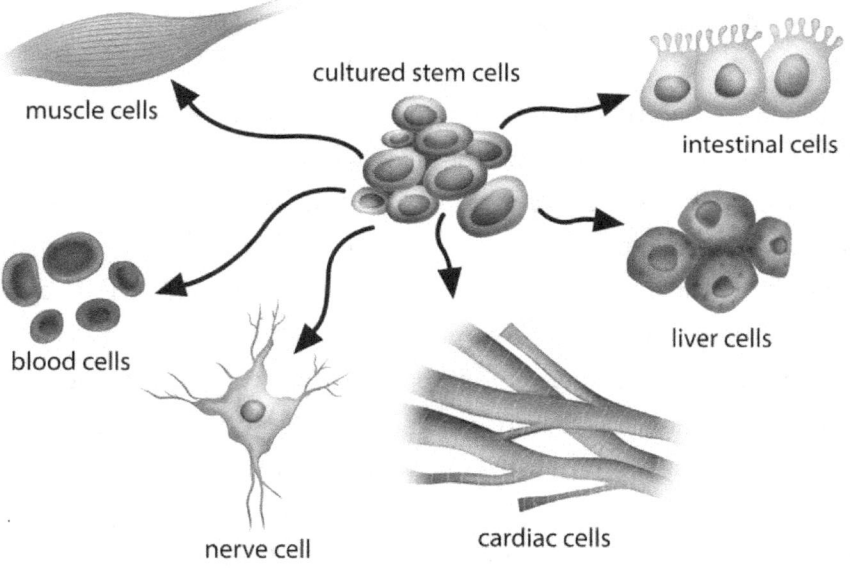

(© blueringmedia - Fotolia.com)

Stem cells are undifferentiated cells that have the ability to become multiple distinct cell types.

These adult stem cells can be used in stem cell therapies as well. The big advantage is that your own stem cells are accepted effortlessly in other parts of your body. The risk of rejection is eliminated. The disadvantage is that these adult stem cells are far less potent than embryonic stem cells. Whereas embryonic stem cells are pluripotent, adult stem cells are multi-potent and can produce only a limited number of cell types.

The use of stem cells offers exciting new possibilities to treat diseases that involve degeneration or destruction of cells. In Spain, for example, researchers have successfully made adult stem cells specialise into cells for the trachea. A piece of trachea, grown in the laboratory, could be implanted into a woman whose trachea had collapsed due to tuberculosis.

Fight

The brain also contains stem cells, but research into these cells is still in an early stage. New neurones appear to originate from glial cells, the cells that populate our brains together with the neurones. In contrast to neurones, glia are able to divide and multiply. The astrocyte is the most occurring glial cell. A special type of astrocyte exists: a mother cell or stem cell. They can develop into ordinary astrocytes, but can also become neurones.

Many of the new-born neurones die rapidly, because they don't get enough support to reach adulthood. Our brain environment is harsh and it is not easy to survive there. Cells have to fight to get the substances they need to grow. These substances are scarce. The strongest and thus the best cells will triumph.

Only a small part of the new brain cells will succeed in

growing up to become adult neurones. This process takes about two months. Then the new neurone will migrate into brain regions where they are needed. There they will be assigned a task in one of the networks.

Neurogenesis is one of the first processes to come to a halt when problems arise within the brain. Chronic stress and diseases obstruct the birth of new neurones. On the other hand, activities also exist that will promote neurogenesis (more on this in chapters 12 and 13).

Apart from the hippocampus one other area exists in the adult brain of which we are sure new neurones come into being. This area is located next to the lateral ventricles of the ventricular system. The new neurones born here have a special task. They migrate to the nerve centre of our sense of smell, which is located in the brain right behind the nose. The neurones in the olfactory bulb, as this area is called, are unique. They are the only ones with a direct connection to the outside world via our noses. They are easily affected due to this direct exposure to the environment. That's why they have a constant cycle of birth, development, and death. Olfactory neurones are replaced every one to two months throughout adulthood.

A constant influx of new neurones is indispensable for our sense of smell. A decline in olfaction may be the first sign of trouble within the brain. It is also one of the possible symptoms of dementia. After all, problems in the brain may cause a glitch in neurogenesis. And without a sufficient supply of new neurones the olfactory bulb cannot function properly anymore.

Stem cells appear to dwell as well in the mucous membrane that lines the inside of our noses. These cells can easily be harvested and thus offer good possibilities for stem cell therapy.

Maybe it's a good idea to think about this for a moment next time you are casually picking your nose.

8. CHAIN REACTION

What is going on in a demented brain?

Of course, we all hope to get old as healthy and physically fit as possible. The normal human ageing process does not prevent this from happening. In general, a mild decline in cognitive abilities occurs. People past seventy mostly aren't as fast and sharp anymore as when they were thirty.

But a reduction in certain kinds of mental agility is countered by an increase in knowledge gained in the course of experience. As for memory and learning, with repetition and enough additional practice recall by older people will equal that by younger. Nor do they forget learned material more rapidly. Problems in the elderly arise due to a lack of concentration and because not enough time is spent learning new facts, but they are not caused by an inability to learn and remember.

Physiological changes accompany growing older. Gradual declines occur in muscular strength and flexibility. A slight change in aimed movements may happen and it may take more time to launch a motion.

As for bodily sensibility, with age there seems to be a reduction in sensitivity to vibration and pain and some loss of sensitivity to detection of fine movements of various joints. Certain reductions occur in the efficiency of seeing, mainly in the ability to focus on nearby objects. We have to buy glasses to be able to see well at short distance and those glasses have to become stronger over time.

In our modern, rather noisy environment a progressive decline in the ability to hear higher frequencies of sound takes place. Some decay in tasting and smelling may happen. Fortunately, the perception of sour and bitter odours diminishes first, whereas pleasant smells such as sweetness remain longest.

One in three people over 75 years of age, who do not suffer dementia, do complain about memory deficits. A slight decline in memory functioning is still considered part of normal ageing. This mainly concerns saving new information. Storing this new information is often done inefficiently, without paying attention. This makes the information hard to recall later on.

Cognitive decline in normal ageing is not caused by a loss of neurones. It is brought about by a decrease in the number of synaptic connections and a loss of neuromodulation. Speed of performance becomes slower, possibly due to ageing neural networks. Connections get weaker or broken with age. The brain has to work harder and longer to find an alternative neural route.

All in all, a wide variability exists in the rate and severity of cognitive decline with age. This is certainly true for personal perception. Where personality is concerned, old age is a revealing time. The best and worst stand out from personality traits present throughout life. Some become self-centred and only concentrate on their ailments. Others accept their restrictions and welcome new opportunities to lead an interesting life.

Decline
This becomes so much more difficult if grave illnesses

happen. In such situations, the ageing process can be accompanied by substantial decline. Then dementia is the phantom that dominates thought. There's so much talk about dementia nowadays that getting older almost appears synonymous to becoming demented.

The fact that dementia seems to be far more common now isn't only because we know a lot more about dementia, but also because people are reaching more advanced ages. With increased age, people run increased risk to suffer dementia. In the past, people died before they reached the ages at which they could start losing their cognitive abilities. With life expectancy increasing, the number of elderly who suffer dementia will grow further the coming decades.

Certainly not everybody reaching their eighties or nineties will experience serious cognitive decline ending in dementia. Different studies come up with different percentages and numbers are certainly different for different parts of the world.

In India for example dementia is relatively rare among its elderly population. Among other things this might have to do with what people in India eat (more on this in chapter 11). It looks as though a quarter of people over eighty years of age in the developed Western world suffer a certain degree of dementia.

Dementia isn't an illness by itself. It is a cluster of behavioural symptoms and is caused by underlying processes. Over fifty causes and diseases have been indicted for generating dementia.

The most well-known is Alzheimer disease. Others are for instance stroke, Parkinson disease, and other neurodegenerative diseases. Also alcoholism, infections such as AIDS and syphilis, brain tumours, toxic exposure, head injury, and a vitamin B12 deficiency may lead to dementia syndrome.

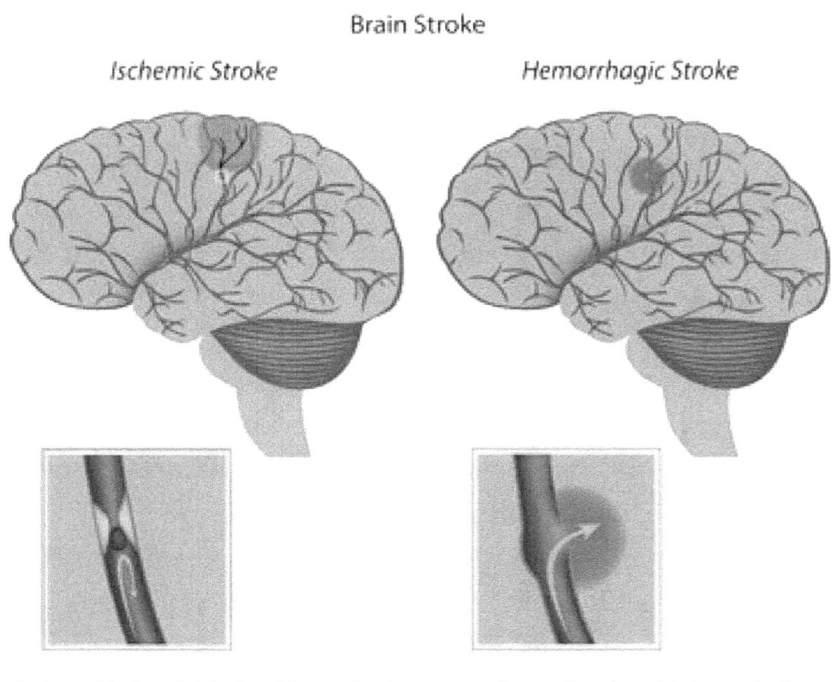

Brain Stroke

Ischemic Stroke   *Hemorrhagic Stroke*

Blockage of blood vessels: lack of blood flow to affected area   Rupture of blood vessels: leakage of blood

(© Alila Medical Media – Fotolia.com)

Brain stroke is one of the over fifty causes and diseases that have been indicted for generating dementia.

Dementia is a clinical syndrome that involves loss of memory and cognitive impairments of sufficient severity to interfere with social or occupational functioning. At least two abnormalities need to be present for someone to be diagnosed with dementia. There has to be memory loss in an otherwise alert patient and the person has to have impairment in at least one other area of cognition such as language, problem solving, judgment, calculation, attention, or perception. Motor skills are little impaired in dementia. In the last stages of the syndrome, basic personality and social skills are affected.

In exceptional cases, dementia is static or even reversible. This is for example the case if the dementia is caused by a malfunctioning thyroid. When the patient receives medicines to correct the thyroid problem the dementia symptoms will disappear as well. Dementia brought about by a vitamin B12 deficit can also be curbed. Administering of vitamin B12 will halt further atrophy of the brain.

Many elderly experience depressions. These sometimes coincide with a decline in cognitive abilities. This is called pseudo-dementia. Treatment with antidepressants not only controls the depression, but also the dementia symptoms. Unfortunately, antidepressants can also have a negative effect on cognition, just like other drugs elderly use to take frequently, like sleeping pills and tranquillisers.

Mystery

Most types of dementia start a chain reaction of irrevocable decline. No cure exists yet, although there are treatments that could ease certain symptoms. As said before, Alzheimer disease is the most well-known and the most common cause of dementia. In laboratories worldwide, researchers are frenetically trying to find ways to prevent and cure this disease.

Sadly, obscurity still surrounds the disease named after the German psychiatrist Alois Alzheimer, the first one to describe the symptoms of the disease at the beginning of the last century. It is even hard to determine whether someone suffers Alzheimer disease. No test is available yet to definitely establish the diagnosis. Only brain biopsy after death can give an unambiguous answer. The diagnosis Alzheimer disease is given after all kinds of tests and examinations have excluded other types of dementia. Based on the presence of specific waste products in the cerebrospinal fluid drained via a spinal tap, specialists today can make a fairly accurate prediction.

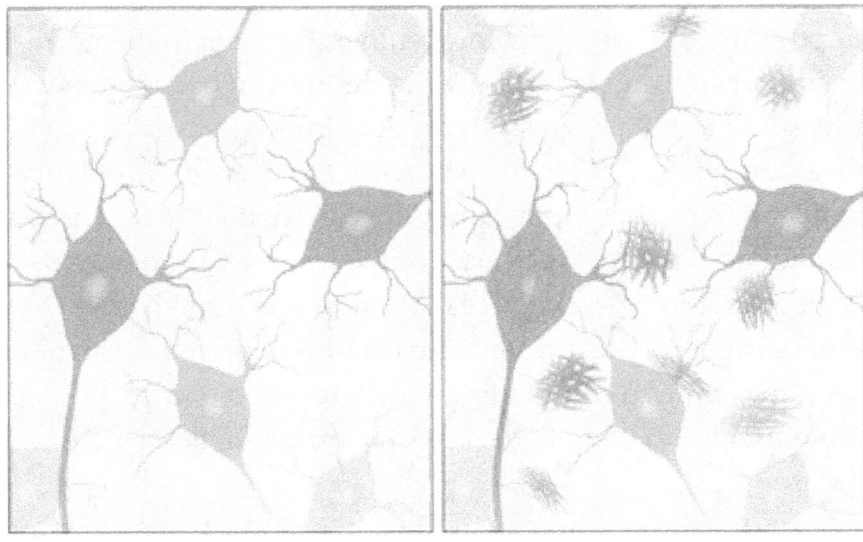

Healthy   Alzheimer's

One of the physical signs of Alzheimer disease are senile plaques, clumps of insoluble protein between neurones.

The causes of Alzheimer disease remain a mystery. In about ten percent of patients, the disease is clearly linked to a genetic deficiency. In the rest no identifiable genetic component has been found yet.

Dietary and other environmental risk factors related to culture seem to influence the incidence of the disease. Alzheimer disease is more common in Europe and the United States, whereas people in Asia suffer more from vascular dementia, caused by strokes.

The risk of contracting Alzheimer disease increases with age, but it definitely is not a part of normal ageing. The hippocampus is, as said before, vulnerable even in the normal ageing process and is certainly the first victim of Alzheimer disease. With the progression of Alzheimer disease the hippocampus becomes smaller, hence the memory problems. People with thicker hippocampi develop dementia to a lesser extent. Possibly they have a cognitive reserve to compensate for neuropathological changes. It is not clear yet whether this reserve capacity was present at birth or is acquired during life through cognitive stimulation. Low education and a monotonous job seem to be a risk factor for Alzheimer disease.

Cells in the hippocampus that die don't send signals anymore to their connections in other brain regions. Gradually, they will die too affecting again other cells that will be deprived of their input as well. This is the chain reaction that brings about the process of degeneration characteristic of Alzheimer disease. It involves progressively worsening memory, language and visuospatial skills, and changes in personality. This process may take from ten to twelve years and will lead to the death of the patient.

Waste

Alzheimer disease is a neurodegenerative disease. This type of disorders is associated with disruptions in the performance of neurones and their death. Neurones are very sensitive to a lack of oxygen. While ageing, the cerebral blood flow tends to show a progressive decline, among other things due to hardening of blood vessels. Less oxygen is reaching the brain, which results in disturbances in neuronal metabolism. Glial cells will come to the aid of distressed neurones. It has in fact been ascertained that these glial cells are far more active in the older brain.

But sometimes these glia go too far in their urge to help neurones. They consider the waste products resulting from the disrupted metabolism dangerous intruders and start an attack. They produce chemicals to destroy the intruders. In large quantities these chemicals are toxic to neurones. The good intentions of the glia achieve exactly the opposite and cause the death of neurones. This is often the case in neurodegenerative diseases.

This kind of aggressive reaction of glial cells can also be aroused by a surplus of insulin in the brain. Insulin helps neurones to absorb glucose, a sugar that serves as fuel for the tiny energy factories inside neurones. If for any reason the insulin cannot make contact with a neurone it will stay behind in the space between cells and will pile up there. This is for instance the case in elderly who suffer type 2 diabetes.

The surplus of insulin could also cause a fierce response of glial cells. Their attack could again result in the death of neurones. Besides, neurones could end up with a fuel shortage since the insulin isn't helping them to absorb glucose. They starve, so to say. In the brains of people with

Alzheimer disease a surplus of insulin that wasn't able to make contact with neurones indeed has been shown.

One of the avenues researchers look for a cure for Alzheimer disease are these overzealous glial cells. If they would succeed in keeping these under control it might be possible to stop or even prevent the domino effect of dying neurones.

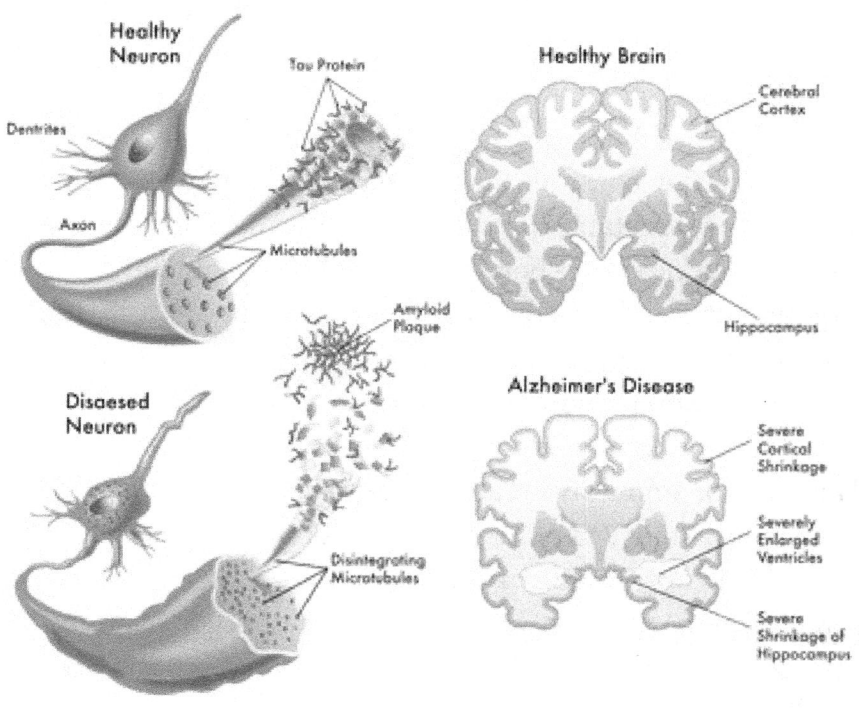

© rob3000

Alzheimer disease is characterised by a chain reaction of cells dying, which results in a process of degeneration. This involves progressively worsening memory, language and visuospatial skills, and changes in personality.

The most characteristic physical signs of Alzheimer disease in the brain are tangles and senile plaques. Tangles are knots of protein fibres within neurones and senile plaques are clumps of insoluble protein between neurones.

It is not known yet why these tangles and plaques appear. For one reason or another, the production of the proteins concerned goes awry. Also in the brains of elderly people who didn't suffer dementia when they died, some tangles and plaques are present only far less than in the brains of Alzheimer's patients.

The plaques and tangles first occur in the brain area where the hippocampus is also situated. They are to blame for the disruption of the connections to memory systems. A diligent search is on for medicines that could help dissolve the abundant tangles and plaques or even prevent them from emerging.

Genetic

This takes us back to the introduction of this part of the book: our genes and to what degree they determine our lives. Alzheimer disease is one of the most intensively researched diseases of recent date.

Very little is known yet about the relationship between this disease and our genes.

In a small number of cases of Alzheimer disease, a hereditary factor is obvious since the disease runs in families. In these cases, people are often stricken by the disease well before they turn 65 years of age. This type of Alzheimer disease is indicated as early-onset Alzheimer disease. Mutations in a few genes have already been found that contribute to early-onset Alzheimer's.

The more common type of Alzheimer disease that presents itself at later age, in most cases cannot directly be linked to hereditary factors within a family. But its cause may lie in gene variants.

As stated above, genes direct the production of proteins. Alzheimer disease is characterised by among other things proteins that become entangled and form clumps. Thus something has to be wrong in the genes that control the production of these specific proteins. In fact, indications have been found that support this idea.

A genetic link has also been found for the fact that far more women than men suffer Alzheimer disease. Let's first cite biology class: the 23rd pair of chromosomes in every human cell comprises the sex chromosomes. If this 23rd pair consists of two X-chromosomes the owner will then be of the female sex. In men, the 23rd pair is formed by an X and a Y-chromosome.

According to a recent study, a gene variant on both X-chromosomes in women could increase the risk of developing Alzheimer disease.

But the most practical explanation of the more frequent incidence of Alzheimer disease in women is of course that women in general live longer than men and thus are more at risk, since the chance to suffer dementia increases with age.

In years to come, surely more genes will be discovered that play a part in the development of Alzheimer disease or that on the contrary offer protection against the disease.

But although cautious preliminary conclusions have been drawn about genetic influence on the development of Alzheimer's, no doubt exists of course that these genes first have to be activated before the degeneration process starts that finally will result in Alzheimer disease. Environmental factors, like diet, living conditions, and lifestyle, will most certainly turn out to play a part of utmost importance.

PART III A BETTER BRAIN

Actually, no reasons exist why you should not possess a well-functioning brain until very advanced age. While the human brain developed over the course of time, many ingenious devices came into being to protect it: a hard skull, the blood-brain barrier, intricate teamwork of brain cells, chemical substances that help cells survive, other substances that destroy dangerous intruders.

If an engineer had to develop a brain machine using an unlimited amount of parts and appliances he would not be able to do so as perfectly as the brain we own today thanks to the adding, the deleting, and the fine-tuning during hundreds of thousands of years of evolution.

Despite all the precautionary measures, brains falter from time to time. They are stricken by disease and lose part of their abilities. When we weren't getting older than about forty or fifty years we hardly noticed anything of these problems. Notwithstanding certain defects our brains kept going until the moment of death.

At the present time, we are growing older and older and the brain may break down long before the end of our lives. With the growing number of years, the number of problems within the brain may increase as well. Until time comes when all these shortcomings cannot stay hidden anymore and the brain succumbs to dementia.

Fortunately, it is not so that everybody in the end becomes demented if they just live long enough. Many brains do exist that keep on doing what they are supposed to do until very advanced age.

In the meantime we have learned this isn't only owed to the package of genes you received from your parents. The functioning of your brain is especially influenced by your lifestyle. On that score, we really don't take very good care of our brain nowadays. During the past fifty years, we have gradually been exercising less and less; we are exposed to ever more stress; and we eat increasingly unnaturally.

The brain has an amazing ability to protect itself and to adapt. Although this plasticity isn't as substantial in old age as during childhood it still exists. But while ageing, we have to stimulate the brain more to use its powers.

Anyone who wants to give their brain at least a good chance to get old in a healthy way, has to realise some essential adjustments to their way of living.

9. REST AND UNREST

Indispensable sleep and harmful stress

Stress and sleep have one thing in common: too much of it is bad for your health, but too little won't do you good either. Too much stress and too little sleep are the most damaging. Too little arousal and too much sleep on the other hand also exert a negative influence on the brain. You have to get the right amount of both stress and sleep. But this right amount is different for everybody. So it is very important to find out how much stress you need to function optimally and after how many hours of sleep you feel comfortably rested and energetic.

Tension

In our present-day busy lives, stress has become a buzzword. Everybody is under a lot of pressure. Due to everything you want and everything you have to do in your free time and on the job, it is your schedule that keeps control of your life. It is hard to find people who do not feel quite stressed regularly. Stress is defined as a persistent mental strain. Originally, the term stems from the area of physics where stress has to do with mechanical strain that can lead to distortion of a material. The psychological meaning of the word recently became in vogue during the fifties thanks to the work of Hans Selye, a Canadian researcher from Hungarian descent. He defined stress as the process of transactions in which the resources of an organism are matched against the demands of the environment. Is the organism adapting well then it will feel positive stress. When the circumstances are unfavourable and the organism isn't feeling at ease in its surroundings, it experiences negative stress.

Stress is a natural part of life. In human beings, it mainly concerns whether someone feels able to cope with the demands the environment poses. The appraisal of the importance of the demands is different for every individual. One person may flourish under a certain tension while another feels overwhelmed and can't cope with the pressure. A third person in the same situation might be – almost literally – bored to death.

It is clear, stress depends mainly on how someone perceives events and reacts to them. Since it is a subjective concept, stress can also be managed and controlled. A person that succeeds in approaching a stressful situation in a positive and relaxed way will take away a large part of the negative influence.

Positive stress comes from challenging and rewarding activities. A situation can be experienced as challenging. This happens when a person thinks his resources approximate or exceed the demands. Good stress also puts the body under strain, but generally this lasts only a short period and doesn't generate negative consequences on the long run. The bodily reactions mimic aerobic exercise with an increased heart rate and decreased vascular resistance which facilitates an optimal blood flow. At an optimal level of stress, the brain is moderately aroused. All your resources are mobilised and full attention is given to the surroundings. You are emotionally balanced and are giving your best performance.

Negative stress arises when situations are experienced as

threatening. Heart rate increases, but vascular resistance does not decrease. This results in an increase in blood pressure and will cause serious health problems in the long term, such as a heart attack or a stroke. Bad stress may also lead to anxiety or depression. Prolonged or severe stress constitutes a serious risk factor for your health. Many of the mental and physical changes caused by stress are similar to those due to infection. Too much stress involves clearly recognisable warning signs. On the emotional level, these are anxiety, apathy, irritability, and mental fatigue. Behaviourally, too much stress leads to avoidance of responsibilities and relationships, extreme or self-destructive behaviour, self-neglect, and poor judgment. Physically, warning signs are excessive worry about illness, physical ailments and complaints, frequent illness, exhaustion, and overuse of medication.

When stress levels are too low, a person becomes inattentive, distractive, and bored.

Survive

Of course, nature has made sure an automated response to stressful situations comes built-in. The most common response is the fight-or-flight response we've talked about before. All body resources are mobilised for a short period to deal with immediate physical dangers. For instance, heart and lungs will work faster; extra nutrients become available for the muscles; pupils will dilate; and metabolism will slow down or stop completely. When the danger has been averted the body soon returns to its normal functioning mode.

This fight-or-flight response has helped man survive in the past when he had to deal with many predators. Evolution made sure the response became ever more sophisticated.

Without it, humans would already have become extinct a very long time ago.

But being able to deal with threats from predators isn't so useful anymore in modern-day life. Still, many contemporary demanding circumstances activate the fight-or-flight response. Activating this system too often or for too long can turn against oneself and become a serious health threat. The body isn't returning to its normal functioning mode. The everyday business of body maintenance is put on hold. This includes the routine tracking down and destruction of foreign or errant cells that could cause diseases.

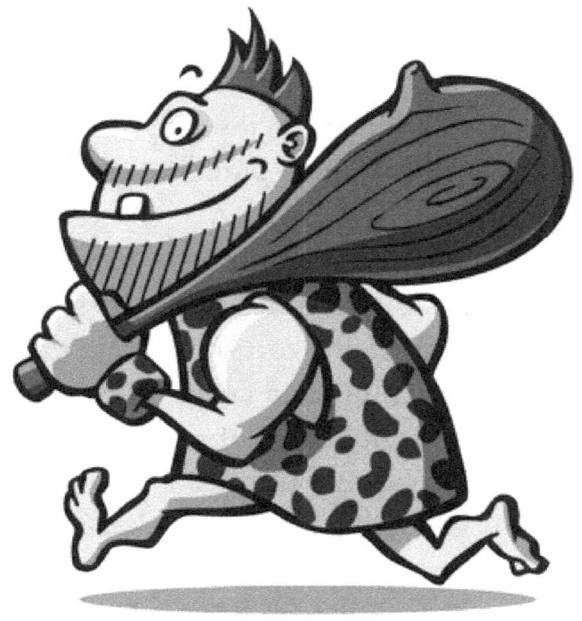

(© pixeldompteur44 - Fotolia.com)

In stressful situations, our bodies are still governed by the fight-or-flight response that helped our ancestors survive when they had to deal with many predators.

Humans nowadays have long-lasting problems, which result in long-term disruption of the body balance. This gives diseases more room to strike. Such a threat does not only come from too much tension, but also from a stimulus under-load when stress levels are too low.

Problems

One part of the brain is particularly sensitive to stress and that is the hippocampus. As we saw, this brain area plays a very important part in learning and memory. While under stress, the body produces the hormone cortisol. This hormone arranges for extra energy to become available to be able to react adequately to a stressful situation. Cells in the hippocampus contain large quantities of receptors for cortisol. If sufficient cortisol has bound to the hippocampal receptors, signals are being sent to another brain area to stop producing the stress hormone.

When the stress is severe and continuous the ability of the hippocampus to do its stress-control job falters. The mechanism to start producing cortisol is being activated again and again. The hippocampus can't cope with the high levels of cortisol and becomes flooded with it. The stress hormones do not damage the hippocampus directly but start a chain reaction that may lead to the death of many neurones. Besides, long-term stress can cause atrophy of dendrites, the small fingers of neurones that have to catch and pass on signals. Stress hormones also influence the prefrontal cortex, the brain's executive area, which is why people often make bad decisions under stress and show increased aggression. Another consequence of stress is that it inhibits the birth of new neurones in the hippocampus. This reduces the volume of the hippocampus. A direct relationship exists between the size of the hippocampus and memory performance. Thus chronic stress leads to impaired memory.

The changes in the hippocampus are reversible as long as the negative stress is terminated after a number of weeks. Longer stress periods result in permanent damage. The cumulative effect of stress starts taking a toll on health in middle age. A connection has also been made between stress in midlife and the development of dementia in late-life. A large group of women in Sweden participated in a 35-year longitudinal population study. Those who reported repeated periods of stress in middle age run a 65 percent higher risk of dementia, mainly from Alzheimer disease, than the ones who did not report repeated periods of stress. So it is a matter of utmost importance to take care of our hippocampus by de-stressing.

Ignitable

Everybody responds differently to stress. Our genes seem to play a role in whether we are more or less sensitive to stress. Researchers have found certain gene variations that make people more reactive to stress. Some stress related disorders are more common in women. This gender bias has a cellular basis. In a specific part of the female brain, cells are more ignitable than in the male brain. These cells activate the response to stress, which thus is more intense in women. In addition, these cells appear to take longer to quiet down again which is why the female brain doesn't adapt swiftly to stressful situations.

In general, a person's response to stress is determined by a combination of genetic, behavioural, and cultural factors. Long-term memory also takes part in the complex process via pleasant or not so pleasant memories from previous stressful situations.

Personal attitudes and coping styles play a significant role. Older people take longer to recover from stress and become less tolerant of strong stressors.

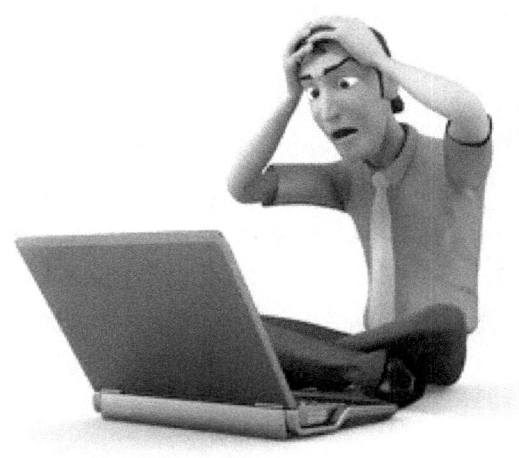

(© CGinspiration - fotolia.com)

A person's response to stress is determined by a combination of genetic, behavioural, and cultural factors. Personal attitudes and coping styles play an important role in recovering from stress.

You can avoid some situations that will make you feel stressed. Noise for example is an obvious stressor, often without you noticing it. Reflect upon the very agreeable silence at the end of the day when all the computers in the office have been turned off. Certain types of music may raise the stress level in your body as well. Even associating with people who are agitated, could influence you negatively.

It is impossible to prevent all tension in your life. That's why it is so important to learn to accept situations you cannot control.

Below are some guidelines that may help you manage the stress in your life:

- First, try to find out what it is that causes stress in your life. Which situations, people or events make you feel nervous or tense?

- Write down when you feel stressed and by what circumstance. Record also how you feel in that circumstance and which physical stress symptoms occur.

- Make your life simpler and prioritise.

- Know your boundaries and learn to say "no".

- Practice to express your thoughts and sentiments.

- Improve your lifestyle, above all where exercise and food are concerned. If you are under a lot of stress for instance, it's better to skip caffeine and other stimulants from your diet. Tranquillisers and alcohol are certainly not the appropriate means to control stress! It would be useful to stop following the news on television, via newspaper or internet for some time. Negative reporting influences your mood and a negative state of mind does contribute to your feelings of pressure.

- Try to find social support. Talking to family and friends is an excellent outlet.

De-stress

Each person has his own ways of coping with stress. Many people do so by engaging in damaging behaviours, such as smoking, drinking alcohol, using drugs, or eating junk food. A diet high in carbohydrates does lower cortisol levels, but the resulting obesity creates more severe health problems. Natural rewards, such as palatable foods, do provide a general means of stress reduction. A study in rats demonstrated that a limited intake of sugary stuff reduces the general stress level. Such a remedy should be used in moderation and with common sense though.

Far healthier ways to dampen stress levels are among other things breathing techniques, yoga, and meditation. For instance, a very simple exercise is to concentrate on your breathing. This will alter your state of consciousness, relaxes, and will detach you from your daily worries. Feel the different types of breathing within your body. Breathe in and out at least eight times as deep, gradually and even as possible. Then go back to your normal respiration. The next step is paying attention to the way you breathe out. Squeeze out as much air as possible and try to exhale just a little longer than the inhalation. When you succeed doing this exercise regularly spread out over the day, it will have an excellent influence on your stress level.

For some relaxation exercises, go lie on your back or sit down in a comfortable way. Pay attention to the different parts of your body. Flex your muscles one by one and go on relaxing them again consciously. You will feel even better when you can picture yourself in beautiful surroundings letting every detail pass in front of your mind's eye.

If you want to go further it may be an option to attend a

course of biofeedback training. Biofeedback will make you conscious of certain bodily functions, such as muscle tone and heart rate. The final goal is to be able to manipulate these bodily functions at will.

Meditation has proven to have extremely positive effects. People who are able to meditate well have lower blood pressure, a lower heart rate, a more even respiration, and improved blood flow. It isn't easy though to reach such a meditative state.

People with a restless mind may benefit from a mantra. A mantra can be a sound, a syllable, a word, or a group of words you repeat silently in your head over and over. This technique bans other, negative thoughts from your mind.

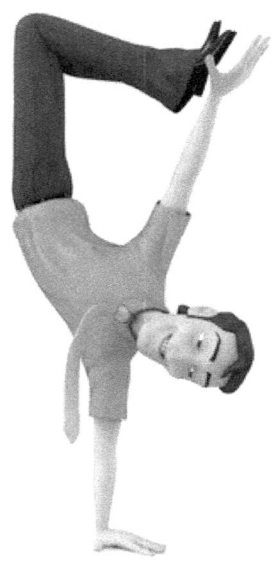

(© CGinspiration - Fotolia.com)

For your long-term health, it is very important to find ways to cope with stress and dampen stress levels.

But of course more plain ways exist to de-stress. Listening to music, taking nature walks, dancing, sports, reading a good book, a massage, and enjoying some kind of hobby all serve the same purpose.

Handling pets is a great stress reliever. Caring for a companion animal not only brings joy and a sense of connection to one's life, it also offers health benefits.

The mere presence of an animal without instruction to attend to it is associated with decreased physiological arousal and decreased anxiety and depression. Stroking a dog or cat increases levels of the hormones that promote nurturing and security and helps boost mood-enhancing neurotransmitters, such as serotonin.

Even looking at a fish in an aquarium relaxes and relieves anxiety for patients sitting in a dental waiting room.

Studies have shown that pet owners, particularly the elderly, have lower blood pressure, are less likely to be depressed and have higher self-esteem than people who don't have pets.

One of the most effective ways to de-stress is laughing. Don't take life too seriously and laugh away your stress. But probably the nicest way to reduce cortisol levels in your body is by making love.

Insomnia

Sleep still is one of the greatest biological mysteries. After many decades of research, we know all about what causes us to feel sleepy, about different types of sleep, about electrical activity in our brains while we sleep, and about the mechanisms of waking up after sleep, but we still don't know why we sleep.

It is clear we do need regular and normal sleep for our overall health. Not sleeping leads to all kinds of problems of which unstable moods are the least damaging. The brain's functioning will also deteriorate due to a lack of sleep. The longer this sleeplessness goes on, the more serious the disruptions become.

Insomnia will eventually cause death. Naturally this last fact hasn't been proven in humans, but in rats. In sleep laboratories, tests are done with human volunteers who are kept awake for a certain period.

Also in torture practices, keeping victims from sleeping has turned out to be an easy and effective way to break their spirit. They literally go crazy.

For our overall health, we regularly do need a certain amount of sleep. And not only us human beings. As far as scientists have been able to test, all animals have some form of periodic sleep. The amount can vary from about three to over twenty hours a day. Even very simple organisms like nematodes and fruit flies sleep.

Some species, for instance the dolphin, have a very peculiar form of sleep. Only one brain hemisphere sleeps at a time. When one hemisphere sleeps the other one can keep an eye on the animal's surroundings and be on the alert for possible predators. Or the waking hemisphere can make sure the owner of the brain surfaces from time to time to catch a breath of fresh air, as in the case of the dolphin.

Birds even have the ability to keep on flying in their sleep driven by their waking hemisphere.

It's a pity we humans didn't develop the ability to continue in our sleep using our waking hemisphere with all those nice things we were doing. We just sleep away one third of our lives.

Types

Sleep obeys the same rules as stress: you shouldn't get too little of it, but neither too much. Individual sleep needs differ. Total sleep time in adults varies between six and nine hours, but in general should be between seven and eight hours. You know your sleep time and sleep quality are adequate when you don't suffer daytime sleepiness or dysfunction

Not only is your sleep time important, but also the quality of your sleep. Some people do sleep enough hours, but still feel sleepy when they get out of bed. This is a sign something is wrong with the way in which they sleep. Maybe the mattress isn't right or the room is too warm. Problems with metabolism could also cause sleep disturbance or sleep disorders.

Sleep is an altered state of consciousness. The brain still processes information. It is aware of the environment and it is controlling body movements. These movements are reduced though, as is the response to stimulation from outside.

Humans go through two types of sleep: rapid eye movement (REM) sleep and non-REM sleep. During REM sleep the eyes make rapid movements and this doesn't happen during non-REM sleep. Non-REM sleep comprises four stages with different electrical activity in the brain. Stages 3 and 4 are the most profound type of sleep. During non-REM sleep neuronal activity is low. Metabolic rate and brain temperature are at its lowest.

REM sleep is a more active form of sleep. Most neurones are just as active as during wakefulness. The brain keeps the body in an immobilised state however. If you suddenly wake up during REM sleep it may feel like an arm or a leg is paralysed. During the night, non-REM and REM sleep alternate. A complete cycle takes between 90 and 110 minutes, which is repeated four to six times a night. The process from stage 1 to 4 is intermittently interrupted by body movements and partial arousals. The length of REM sleep increases while the night advances and sleep stages 3 and 4 decrease.

Catching up
Sleep is strictly regulated. Sleep loss is inevitably followed by a rebound. This catching up sleep is more efficient than normal sleep. It consists of more REM sleep and more deep sleep.

The exception to this sleep rule is a group of people who suffer a unique disease called fatal familial insomnia. This is an inheritable disease. It runs in only about forty families worldwide. Sufferers carry a gene mutation that manifests itself usually between 35 and 60 years of age. The persons concerned are troubled with increasing insomnia due to which they generally will die within one to three years. The first registered victim of the disease was an Italian who died in 1765. Unknowingly, the disease has been passed on for centuries from generation to generation. Finally, in the nineties of the last century, fatal familial insomnia has been recognised as an inheritable affliction and could be deduced to a genetic aberration. In the future, gene therapy has to give the carriers of this gene hope for a cure.

Although sleep will catch up with us long before we would succumb to insomnia, chronic sleep deprivation does have serious consequences for our health. The body's production of stress hormones rises with all the damaging results mentioned before.

All kinds of chemical processes in the body are disrupted. Blood pressure rises. Chronic sleep deprivation is linked to serious diseases such as heart disease, psychosis, anxiety disorders and depression.

Recent research even showed that people, who don't sleep enough, become more obese. Sleep deprivation may disrupt hormones that regulate glucose metabolism and appetite. Less sleep results in higher levels of an appetite-stimulating hormone, and lower levels of an appetite-suppressing hormone.

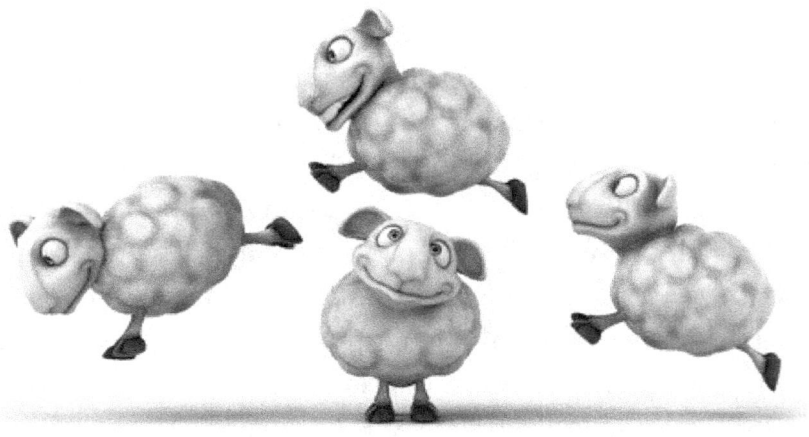

(© julien tromeur - Fotolia.com)

Sleep deprivation is possibly the biggest enemy of good health. Chronic sleep deprivation is linked to serious diseases and even such a thing as fatal insomnia exists. Our immune system needs sleep to recover.

Benefits
It is clearly beneficial to us to spend a certain amount of hours in a sleeping state every day. But we still don't know why we need to sleep. Apparently, some benefits emerge from the

environmental disconnection sleep produces that cannot be provided by quiet wakefulness. A few discoveries have been made that give some insight. Sleep is largely under genetic control. It can serve many functions or just one, until now unknown function. Several theories on the mystery of sleep have been proposed.

It is a fact that the immune system that has to protect us against disease is positively influenced by sleep. Researchers counted the number of white blood cells, the building blocks of our immune system, in various mammalian species. The more total hours of sleep a species enjoys, the higher their number of white blood cells. Sleep deprivation in rats on the other hand showed a twenty percent decrease in their number of white blood cells.

A sleeping period probably is also useful to give the body time to recover from the activities during the day and return all the processes to their normal mode. During wakefulness, many processes are pushed to their maximum levels. During non-REM sleep various organs appear to be recovering from the pressure during the day. Many brain networks do the same during REM sleep. When we sleep, a lot of clearing up and repair activities are taking place in our brain. That's why many of the symptoms of a shortage of sleep resemble signs of overload.

Everybody does agree by now sleep plays an essential part in the performance of our memory. Many studies have shown that while sleeping the brain is busy consolidating memories. Evidence for this feat came from research in rats of which brain activity was measured. First, the rats had to learn something, for instance finding their way through a maze to get to some food. While they were mastering this task certain parts of their brains were active. Afterwards the rats went to sleep. During that sleeping period the same brain parts became active in the same way as when they were learning. It was as if the rat brain again went through what was learned step by step while sleeping.

The most important brain area for this task of course is again the hippocampus. This area turns out to be especially active during REM sleep. This made scientists come to the conclusion that REM sleep is important for the consolidation of memories. A lack of REM sleep results in an increase in the stress hormone cortisol and a decrease in new neurones. And that is bad news for the hippocampus and for our memory.

So it is a good idea to go to sleep right after having learned something you need to remember well. But no scientific evidence exists it may be useful to put your textbooks under your pillow.

Pattern

With increasing age, sleep patterns change. Above all, the amount of REM sleep declines. In new-borns, it constitutes about 50 percent of total sleep, whereas in elderly people only 15 to 20 percent of total sleep is REM sleep. This may be due to the fact that REM sleep promotes the development of brain circuits for learning and thus may be far more important for the developing brain. Babies learn a lot of new things that have to be stored in memory.

Deep sleep, stage 3 and 4 of non-REM sleep, also decreases gradually. This can have serious consequences since it is important as restorative sleep. During deep sleep the immune system is being recharged. A faltering immune system results in susceptibility to all kinds of diseases.

The amount of sleep we need remains fairly constant throughout our lives. Older people rarely get the sleep they need since they generally sleep more lightly. Besides, their nocturnal sleep is interrupted by many short awakenings. Many elderly have problems falling asleep, staying asleep, and falling back to sleep. About half of older adults suffer from insomnia.

This can have worrying effects. Consequences of insufficient sleep in the elderly may be cognitive decline, increased risk of falls, daytime fatigue, and reduced physical and mental health. Disordered sleep is a major problem in people with dementia, as their sleep/wake cycles are drastically altered. Chronic sleep deprivation may even contribute to the build-up of plaques in the brain, an excess of which are seen in Alzheimer disease.

Routine

It is clear a good night's sleep is extremely important in keeping your brain healthy into very old age. Many remedies may help counteract insomnia. Complete books have been written about it. I name just a few examples: avoid stimulants such as coffee and cigarettes shortly before going to bed. Alcohol is not a stimulant, but it does impair sleep quality as it limits REM sleep. Certain food additives also interfere with sleep as does a large evening meal. Don't exercise late in the evening. The amount of time between exercising and going to bed should be at least four hours.

It is wise to stick to the same bedtime hours every day. A certain degree of daily routine appears to be useful as well in counteracting sleeplessness. Changes in their biological clock could be a cause of insomnia in elderly people. This biological clock among other things regulates your sleep/wake cycle. It makes you feel sleepy so you'll go to bed and after several hours of sleep it wakes you up again. A constant and organised lifestyle may moderate the sleep effects of age-related changes in the biological clock.

The hormone melatonin is very important in the functioning of our biological clocks. If it gets darker, more melatonin is released and you will start to feel sleepy. In the morning, at first light, melatonin production is stopped and you will awake. That's why it so hard to get out of bed early in winter. It is dark outside and melatonin production is still going on. If your biological clock isn't functioning well it is important to remain in areas with bright light during the day. A marked difference between day and night - that is between light and dark - improves the action of the biological clock.

The temperature of the room in which you sleep also is vital for your sleep quality. In a group of people who suffered chronic insomnia an experiment was done placing a cooling cap on their heads during sleep. Researchers had registered faster metabolism in the frontal lobes of the brain in people with insomnia. Normally, metabolism slows down during sleep. Cooling is a method to actively slow down metabolism. So the participants in the experiment had a cap placed on their heads with small tubes incorporated. Cold water flowed through these tubes. This lowered the temperature around the front of their head to about fourteen degrees Celsius. Thanks to this cooling, the insomnia sufferers slept just as well as the people in a control group that did not suffer sleeplessness. The cooling cap even had another positive effect since it made the persons using it spend more time in the very healthy, deep sleep part of the sleep cycle.

More research has to be done on the effect of cooling on sleep, but this experiment is a scientific confirmation of what we actually already knew: that a cool room is critical to a good night's sleep.

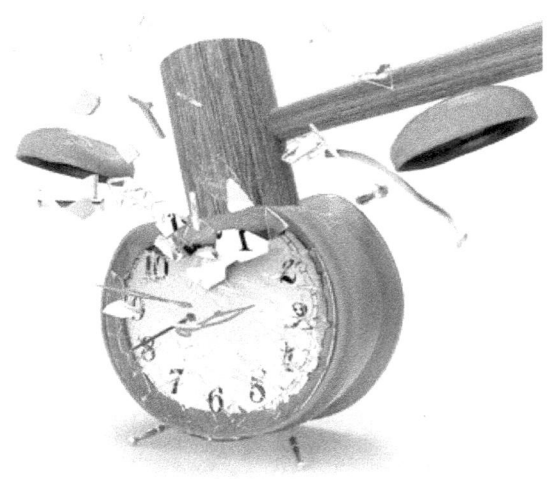

(© Haver - Fotolia.com)

Make sure you go to bed on time and sleep the sufficient amount of hours so you'll wake up spontaneously, without the need for an alarm clock.

Alarm clock

Insomnia has many different causes: stress, noise, medicines, hormones, depression, or pain. If you have trouble falling asleep don't seek refuge in sleeping pills right away. Start with natural ways to attack the sleeplessness:

- Go to bed at about the same time every day and do the same with getting out of bed, also during weekends.

- Create a fixed bedtime routine. A sequence of activities like brushing your teeth, undressing, and assuming your favourite sleeping position, constitutes a signal for your brain it is time to go to sleep. You can even extend your routine with other activities like taking a short walk, taking a warm bath, meditating, or performing relaxation exercises.

- Make sure you get enough physical activity during the day and try to spend some time outside every day, in natural light.

- A siesta is good for you, but it shouldn't last too long. Limit an afternoon nap to no more than ten to twenty minutes so it doesn't affect your night-time sleep negatively.

- Learn to relax, for instance via breathing exercises, meditation, or yoga. When you have a very active mind, it may bring relief if you concentrate on a certain image like the sun or a flower, or a specific word and focus all your attention on it. This will help you chase off other thoughts. Above all, don't worry about the fact that you are not able to fall asleep since that will surely keep you awake.

- To get the production of melatonin going, it is a good idea to dim all the lights in your home about an hour before your bedtime. If your family members complain, put on sun glasses for the same effect.

- If you wake up frequently during the night you may not have the right type of bed. Possibly your mattress is too hard or too soft; your bed base may be worn out; or your pillow may not give sufficient support. If you awaken regularly because you have to urinate be sure not to drink coffee and alcohol in the evening.

- If you are a light sleeper and wake up easily or when you have to sleep in a noisy environment you could try a white noise machine. Such a device produces a soothing, relaxing sound, such as of a breeze, the surf, or a waterfall, to drown the disturbing noise.

- When you stay awake for too long, get up and do something relaxing, like reading. After a short while, go back to bed and try again to fall asleep.

In the next chapters, you will find information about how you can stimulate the two most important stages of the sleep pattern, REM sleep and deep sleep.

In our society, sleep is often seen as a waste of time. People who need little sleep (or at least claim that they do) are being admired. In television series about hospitals and emergency rooms, the sleepless nights of the resident physicians are being romanticised, whereas in reality a lack of sleep can lead to serious mistakes with dramatic consequences.

Try not to see sleep time as a necessary evil, but instead as a pleasant activity that is very healthy as well. And if possible, throw that alarm clock into the garbage bin. Go to bed at the right time and wake up spontaneously in the morning when you are done sleeping. After all, you don't turn on the alarm clock to make you cease other enjoyable activities in life, such as making love or eating?!

10. ENJOY YOUR MEAL

Healthy eating comes in many variations

Eating is a matter of life-and-death. On the other hand, if you eat the wrong kinds of food you could also die. The views on which kind of foods are good for our bodies and which ones can cause damage are worlds apart. The ideas about what you should and what you should not eat change radically in the course of time. In the past, milk appeared an indispensable part of our diet. Nowadays, there is a growing body of opinion that milk actually isn't so healthy for us, with the exception of mother's milk. Whereas sweetener seemed to be the solution to avoid the use of sugar with all its calories, it is now clear that certain sweeteners play an obvious role in the development of cancer.

Through the years, an awful lot of foodstuffs have been linked to the development of cancer. At one point in time, you weren't even allowed to scrape the last bit of diet margarine from its tub since the tiny plastic parts that thus would enter your body could also result in cancer.

Fortunately, today we are a bit more down-to-earth and news about another ingredient in our food that might cause cancer isn't reaching the media every week anymore. It is a fact though that all those complicated processes in the factory do not make food healthier. The more foodstuffs are treated, for instance to make them less perishable, the bigger the chance of losing healthy vitamins and minerals and of adding possibly dangerous chemical substances.

As pure as possible, fresh and raw are words that go with healthy eating. If you have the possibility, 'unsprayed' and 'free-range meat' chip in as well.

Satisfying

You are what you eat. Of course your hair won't turn orange because you eat a lot of carrots. But everything that enters your body via your food does have a direct influence on the structure and the functioning of the cells in your body. They live on the substances within the food you eat. Improper diet is clearly linked with disease and premature ageing. Centenarians all have their own recipe for a long and healthy life. They may have a wide variety of diets, but they have one thing in common: they eat moderately and generally maintain a constant weight.

An important aspect of a healthy diet is that it not only has to provide a balanced supply of nutrients several times a day, but has to be psychologically satisfying as well. When you force yourself to eat all kinds of healthy foods that you actually don't like it won't produce the desired results. Generally speaking, a healthy diet consists of the appropriate amounts of all nutrients and an adequate amount of water. There should be a balance of macronutrients and micronutrients. Macronutrients are carbohydrates, fats, and proteins. They are needed in large amounts and provide energy. Food is digested in the gastrointestinal tract and generates three types of energy. Lipids are formed from fat, amino acids from protein, and glucose from carbohydrates. Most foods contain all three forms of macronutrients. Micronutrients are minerals and vitamins. They are needed in smaller quantities.

Metabolism is the chemical process by which food is converted into energy. This energy is used to run and repair the body.

What we eat also has a big influence on our brain. The brain consumes no less than 25 percent of the glucose that enters our body. Glucose is made out of carbohydrates. Our cells use it as fuel to keep their machinery going.

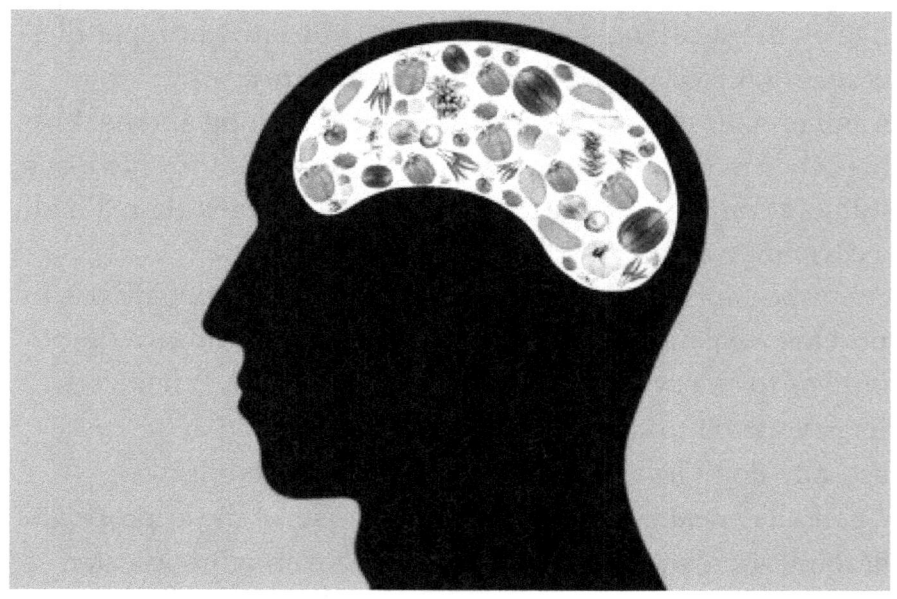

(© meepoohyaphoto - Fotolia.com)

The brain is greatly influenced by what we eat since it consumes 25 percent of the fuel that enters our body via our food. What we eat is also fundamental to how we think and feel.

What's more, our food is fundamental to how we think and feel. The nutrients we take in affect the formation and activity of neurotransmitters, the chemicals that transport information from one neurone to the next. Carbohydrates for instance set off a chain reaction for the production of serotonin, the neurotransmitter that is an important player in depression, insomnia, irritability, and feelings of calmness and serenity. This way, poor diet can lead to changes in mood, confusion, memory loss, depression, and mental disorders.

Antioxidants

In general, a healthy diet consists of a wide variety of fresh, unprocessed foods. This works best for growth, maintenance and division of the cells in our body.

During cellular metabolism, radicals can form. These free radicals are unstable molecules that can damage cells. Oxidative stress results from an inability of the body to get rid of these free radicals. It is involved in many diseases. Radicals play a role for example in the development of cancer cells. Antioxidants are chemical compounds that neutralise these free radicals. They are found in many foods, especially fruits and vegetables. As a rule, it is not very helpful to take antioxidants in supplement form. Most of the times, they don't reach the places where they are needed and sometimes, they even exert a negative influence. Vitamin C as antioxidant in pill form for instance generally stays in the bloodstream and in the extracellular fluid. Besides, an overdose of vitamin C on the contrary can cause damage instead of rendering radicals harmless.

Another example is the antioxidant beta-carotene which among other things gives carrots their orange colour. This antioxidant is unsuitable as a dietary supplement. Research showed that people who smoke and take a beta-carotene supplement have a far bigger chance to get lung cancer than smokers who do not take the supplement. Obviously, it is a far better idea to eat a real carrot from time to time!

It is certainly not wise to glut your body with antioxidants by taking pills. It so happens they might deactivate too many radicals. And it is not only bad news where radicals are concerned. According to the specialists, they also have a positive part to play in our body. It appears they are involved in certain defence mechanisms of cells.

To prevent problems there shouldn't be too many radicals around. That is why it is best to come by the necessary amount of antioxidants in a natural way, by eating a variety of colourful, cruciferous, and leafy green vegetables and fruits. In that way, the required balance between antioxidants and radicals will be created as a matter of course.

Pills and food simply are not the same. Dietary supplements go through all kinds of production processes to finally get them on your table as capsules, pills, or powders. Unknown is whether at that moment all the useful ingredients are still active. Apart from that, fruits and vegetables contain a whole range of useful chemicals that together exert the right, positive influence on the body. Isolating some ingredients in the laboratory obviously does not yield the same result as consuming the rich, natural original.

Vitamins

Vitamins are not synthesised by the body, but acquired through the foods we eat. Vegetables and fruits are also the main suppliers of the vitamins our body needs. So far, thirteen vitamins have been universally recognised, although in some countries more chemical compounds are considered vitamins.

Vitamins serve diverse biochemical functions in metabolism, in cell and tissue growth and differentiation, and as antioxidants. In humans, vitamins are water-soluble or fat-soluble. As the water-soluble vitamins are easily excreted from the body via urine, a consistent daily intake is important. The fat-soluble vitamins accumulate in the body, which may lead to hypervitaminosis.

Nutritional deficiencies of certain vitamins can have devastating effects. They can contribute to depression, personality and mood changes, and insomnia.

For our brains, particularly the B vitamins are indispensable. They are related to cognitive performance. Vitamin B12 plays a key role in normal functioning of the nervous system. It is involved in cell metabolism, in DNA synthesis and regulation, in fatty acid synthesis, and in energy production.

Many elderly people suffer a shortage of vitamin B12. The first symptom is reduced speed of information processing. In the end, vitamin B12 shortage may result in dementia. By administering a vitamin B12 supplement, it is possible to undo many of the symptoms.

Vitamin B6 is also vital for cognitive performance. Among other things, it is involved in metabolism of macronutrients and synthesis of neurotransmitters. One of these neurotransmitters is serotonin, which influences our mood and the functioning of our memory. That's why taking vitamin B6 tablets has been shown to relieve symptoms of premenstrual syndrome and depression and improve memory in older adults.

Vitamin B9, better known as folic acid or folate, is essential to numerous bodily functions. It is necessary to synthesise and repair DNA and to produce blood cells. Folic acid appears to reduce the risk of stroke and to improve cognition in the elderly. A shortage of folic acid is relatively common. Too little folic acid can lead to a progressive condition of mental deterioration with accompanying cerebral atrophy. An older brain that contains high levels of folic acid appears to suffer less from the tangles and senile plaques that characterise Alzheimer disease.

Sunbath

Other vitamins play a significant part as well in keeping our brains healthy.

Vitamin C is generally accepted as an antioxidant. As it protects blood vessels it benefits cognitive function in ageing. Vitamin D is not really a vitamin, but a hormone, produced by the body as a result of exposing the skin to the sun. Vitamin D has many roles in regulating brain health. It is involved in calcium regulation; it has anti-oxidative properties; it takes part in immune system regulation; and, last but not least, it enhances neuronal signalling.

It is obvious, too low vitamin D levels are disastrous. Vitamin D deficiency has been recognised as a worldwide health problem. As many as one billion people in the world may be vitamin D deficient, which is a risk factor for many diseases. That so many people suffer vitamin D deficiency is not only caused by the fact that in many parts of the world sunshine does not abound, but also by the fact that information campaigns about the prevention of skin cancer are very successful. People don't dare to sit in the sun anymore. Nevertheless, taking a sunbath is the most effective way to incite the body to synthesise vitamin D. To get enough vitamin D, unprotected daily exposure to the sun of 5 to 15 minutes is sufficient. Such a sunbath gives the body far more vitamin D than you would be able to get via your food or via dietary supplements.

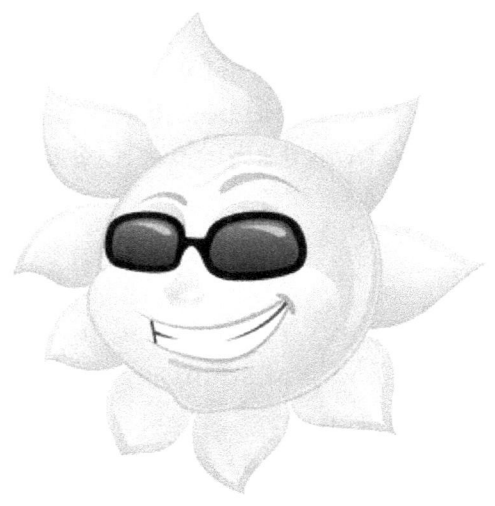

(© Stockerteam – Fotolia.com)

Vitamin D is fundamental to good health. A lack of vitamin D is linked to many diseases. The best way to have your body produce enough vitamin D is exposing your skin to the sun for 5 to 15 minutes daily.

Researchers found vitamin D has a direct influence on over 200 different genes. Vitamin D switches genes on or off. Many of these genes are implicated in disease. That's why a shortage of vitamin D is linked to among others osteoporosis, bone fractures, increased risks of cancers, diabetes, autoimmune diseases, hypertension, stroke, infectious diseases, and psychiatric illnesses. It has been shown for instance a vitamin D deficiency may increase your risk of suffering depression. Older adults are more at risk of a vitamin D deficiency. They usually have a higher fat-to-muscle ratio, which leads to more vitamin D stored in fatty tissue and less available in blood. Besides, older skin is less efficient at making vitamin D from sun bathing. Age-related decline in vitamin D is called hypovitaminosis D (HVD) and possibly as much as 40 percent of older adults suffer from it, thus raising their risk for stroke and dementia.

Supplements

Is it useful to take vitamin supplements? Judging by the huge importance of the different vitamins you would think so. But the answer to this question still isn't clear. No unambiguous answers are given yet to the questions which vitamins to take and how large a dose. In general, ingesting large quantities of vitamins or minerals for longer periods could be harmful and may have adverse health effects.

There certainly exist restraints on the use of certain vitamins. Vitamin E for instance is known for its antioxidant properties. An extra dose of vitamin E however can increase the damage done by free radicals. As a normal diet offers enough vitamin E, it isn't recommended to ingest it as a supplement.

Apart from vitamins, minerals belong to the group of micronutrients as well. Dietary minerals are chemical elements required by all living organisms. Examples of these minerals are potassium, chlorine, sodium, calcium, magnesium, zinc, iodine, and iron. An appropriate intake is necessary to maintain optimal health. Normally, diet can meet these requirements.

Sometimes, you can even get too much of a mineral, voluntarily or involuntarily. This mainly concerns sodium. Not only do we add quite some sodium to our food via the salt shaker, but also nearly all foodstuff coming from the factory contains it. Salt has a slight addictive action. Researchers discovered only half a teaspoonful of salt less per day can work miracles for your health. Your chance of getting cardiovascular diseases diminishes considerably. The effect is comparable to give up smoking. It's useful indeed to search for products in the supermarket that contain less or no added sodium.

Filled up

Our ancestors went out hunting for food when they were hungry. A complicated combined action between the gastrointestinal tract, adipose tissue and the brain results in our feeling hungry. Various hormones enter the brain from our body to indicate the stomach is empty and nutrients are necessary to keep the different body parts running. Then the brain starts actions to come by food. As soon as the stomach has filled up other hormones are sent to the brain to pass on the message there's no need to eat anymore.

This is at least the ideal situation. Unfortunately, the custom to eat when we are hungry is long gone. Our eating habits are governed by very different signals. We don't eat when we are hungry, but at regular mealtimes, whether we have an appetite or not. Eating is also a social activity. Many people complain they eat far more than normal when they take part in an enjoyable dinner with friends. When you see someone eat it makes you want to eat. Watch one of those vivid cooking programs on television. The moment you see the chef put his teeth into a tasty looking dish it makes your mouth water even though you just had a copious dinner.

When and what we eat is influenced by habit. In one part of the world, lunch starts at 12 o'clock, in another part at 2 o'clock. For some people, lunch is the main meal of the day, for other people it's dinner. Also in the evening, the times to be at the table vary largely. North-Europeans like to start their evening meal around 6 o'clock, whereas Argentineans absolutely won't start eating before sunset, which in summer can be close to 10 o'clock. Consequently, due to their full stomachs it's hard for them to fall asleep.

In general, all these variations don't affect our health in a direct way. Breakfast on the other hand is of vital importance for a well-functioning brain. When the body gets going again in the morning after the rest of the night it's only logical it needs fuel.

An investigation in the US revealed that children performed much better at school and showed less behavioural problems after eating a solid breakfast. And it won't be surprising if adults turn out to be able to concentrate more on what they are doing after an extensive breakfast and thus having supplied the brain with fresh glucose.

Acquired tastes also play an important role in our eating habits. Experiences in childhood related to the consumption of food affect our perspective on food consumption later in life. When, for instance, you never ate fish as a child, you can of course force yourself as an adult to regularly eat fish because it is so healthy. But it will never become one of your favourite dishes for which you may be woken up in the middle of the night.

Flavour is a determining factor in human eating behaviour.

Good-tasting food motivates eating. And because it tastes so good we often eat just a little more than would be good for us. Due to our preferences for sugary and fatty foods, a healthy diet is sometimes very difficult to achieve. Sweets often function as mood stabilisers. It is good not to skip them completely from your diet as a sweet every now and then helps to reinforce the correct nutrient intake.

Weight
Weight is an important aspect of health. Overweight and obesity increase the likelihood of various diseases. A new movement in the quest for the fountain of eternal youth is focusing on a calorie restricted diet. Consuming considerably less calories may play a role in improving health and possibly in extending life. This might be related among other things to the fact that brain cells go up the wall a little bit due to a shortage of nutrients. This stress makes brain cells more active and triggers the production of chemical substances that protect brain cells. This extra protection might counteract deterioration of brain cells.

In a wide range of animals, calorie restriction has been shown to slow the ageing process and increase lifespan. To make this happen, the animals are put on a diet containing 30 to 40 percent less calories than normal. Some studies reveal the calorie restricted diet has to be started at a very young age to reach the desired effect. Research is ongoing into the effects of calorie restriction in nonhuman primates and on human health.

In anticipation of the results of this research, some people submit themselves voluntarily to a calorie restricted diet in order to stay young for a longer period and live up to more advanced age. It is by no means certain this approach makes sense. The effect of calorie restriction in humans is controversial. Although some benefits have been demonstrated, side effects such as loss of muscle mass and bone also are extensive. Calorie restriction lowers testosterone levels, which results in reduced libido. It also slows metabolism, which changes thermal regulation. The core body temperature drops and you feel cold more quickly. Besides, by eating very little you may lose out on essential nutrients. Some research studies even came up with opposite results. Low body weight in middle-aged people and elderly appears to be associated with premature mortality risk from cardiovascular disease and cancers. Underweight in people over 65 may generate a higher dementia risk than normal weight or even overweight.

Although obesity in young adulthood and midlife is a big threat to longevity as it results in cardiovascular diseases and diabetes, in older adults a slight overweight seems to be better for health reasons. Over thirteen thousands residents – average age 73 - of a retirement community in the United States took part in a study about weight and mortality. Those who were overweight had the lowest mortality rates.

So it is not really advantageous to starve yourself. A well-balanced, low-fat diet will suit your needs very well. Keep those few pounds of body weight we almost all gain while ageing. As long as you feel comfortable with them.

Menu

In recent times, we have gained a lot of knowledge about the influence of food on our body. All over the world, investigations are taking place into the effects of certain nutrients, targeted specifically towards prevention of diseases. As the interest in healthy diets grows, this results in frequent media coverage of another 'wonder' food which you definitely have to put on your menu in order to stay healthy. Just as often, after a while you don't hear anything anymore about that specific type of fruit or vegetable or the effects don't turn out to be so fantastic in future research.

Below, some of the more established research results of certain foods are highlighted.

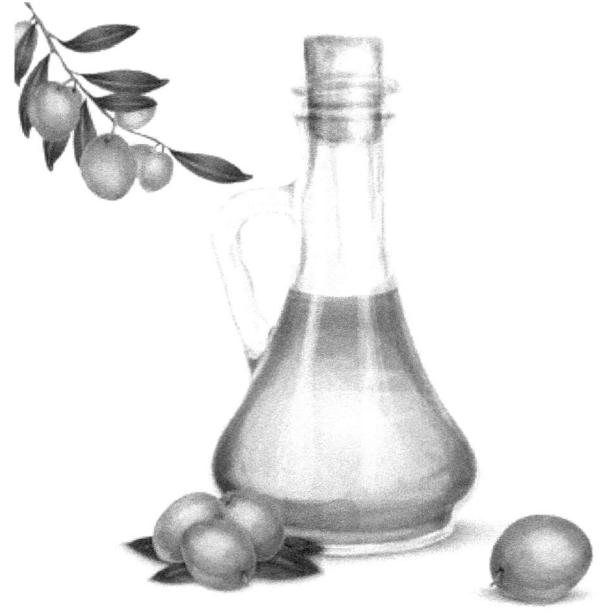

(© macrovector - Fotolia.com)

Extra virgin olive oil is the healthiest type of oil. It doesn't contribute to the amount of radicals in your body, but does provide your cells with the necessary fat to keep their membranes flexible.

A very important food group is the one that contains the previously mentioned antioxidants. These are indispensable to deactivate the excess radicals in our body. One of the ways in which we get a lot of radicals in our body, is by eating food rich in saturated fats, for instance fried foods. Using extra virgin olive oil in preparing your meals is a healthy alternative to other, more damaging oils.

Essentially, all fruits and vegetables hold antioxidants. Very good sources are apples and blueberries. This goes also for broccoli, spinach, potatoes, oranges, and radish. Celery and green peppers contain the substance luteolin, also an antioxidant and good at fighting infections in the brain. Experiments have shown certain foods can directly affect signalling in the brain and neuronal communication. A specific group of chemical substances called polyphenols is involved in this process. More than 4000 polyphenolic compounds have been discovered so far in fruits, vegetables, nuts, seeds, and grains.

They have beneficial effects on infections, allergies, and even cancer, as well as being antioxidants.

Blueberries have become famous in this aspect. They exert a very positive effect on the brain.

Also dark chocolate contains polyphenolic compounds, more specifically the substance called flavonol. This appears to improve blood flow and thus has a positive outcome on learning and memory functions of the brain. But only if it is dark chocolate with a high content of real cacao, preferably at least 80 percent.

The polyphenols found in the skin of red grapes will end up to a certain degree in red wine. Hence the recommendation to drink one glass of red wine every day. Reasonable alcohol intake (one glass a day for women and two glasses a day for men at most) has shown another benefit. It has a relaxing effect on blood vessels, which results in improved cerebral blood flow.

Chronic heavy alcohol ingestion on the other hand has a devastating effect on the brain. It makes neurones shrink and particularly the functioning of the hippocampus is severely disturbed by it. Excessive alcohol use may also increase the risk of brain haemorrhage. In the end, it may lead to dementia.

Drinking alcohol during pregnancy can have serious consequences for the development of the child in the womb. It is for example one of the most frequent causes of mental handicaps at birth in the western world.

Older adults have to be extra careful with regards to their alcohol intake. They have a declining ability to metabolise alcohol and have less water in their body to dilute the alcohol. This makes the alcohol act more rapidly and more intensely in the older brain.

Since we are discussing harmful stimulants, I want to mention the cigarette just once – hopefully unnecessary.

A lot is known about the dangers of smoking. Tobacco addiction is the single greatest cause of preventable illness. Long-term smokers have significantly lower cerebral blood flow. Cigarette smoking damages the brain, but it may take decades before the damage comes to light.

Fuel

Glucose is an important fuel for the brain. It also seems to enhance memory storage. A group of healthy elderly participated in a study to test their memory.

Before taking the test, they were given lemonade with sugar (glucose) and on the next occasion, lemonade with the sugar substitute saccharin. After the glucose drink, they performed far better on memory tests than after the lemonade with saccharin.

Glucose also aids memory retrieval. Students have known this fact for a long time already. They take along some candy to perform better at an exam.

But this doesn't mean it's a good idea to take in a lot of glucose. A high-sugar diet results in low-insulin sensitivity. Insulin, as explained earlier, signals cells to take up glucose from the blood. When insulin sensitivity is low, cells don't get enough signals to take up glucose and will starve.

People with an extra high blood sugar concentration look older. This was revealed by an investigation of a Dutch university. Researchers concluded glucose influences the ageing process of the skin.

Cholesterol ended up with a bad name due to its role in heart disease, but it is an essential ingredient of the body. It is a small organic compound soluble in fat, not in water. The body makes most of its cholesterol from sugars in our diet.

Cholesterol is a component of cell membranes, necessary for membrane permeability and fluidity. The myelin sheath covering neuronal axons is also rich in cholesterol.

In addition, from cholesterol at least five crucial hormones are made. It also contributes to the absorption of fat-soluble vitamins.

The body simply cannot survive without cholesterol. Rapidly lowered cholesterol levels are associated with emotional disorders like depression, anxiety, and panic attacks.

Bad vs. Good Cholesterol

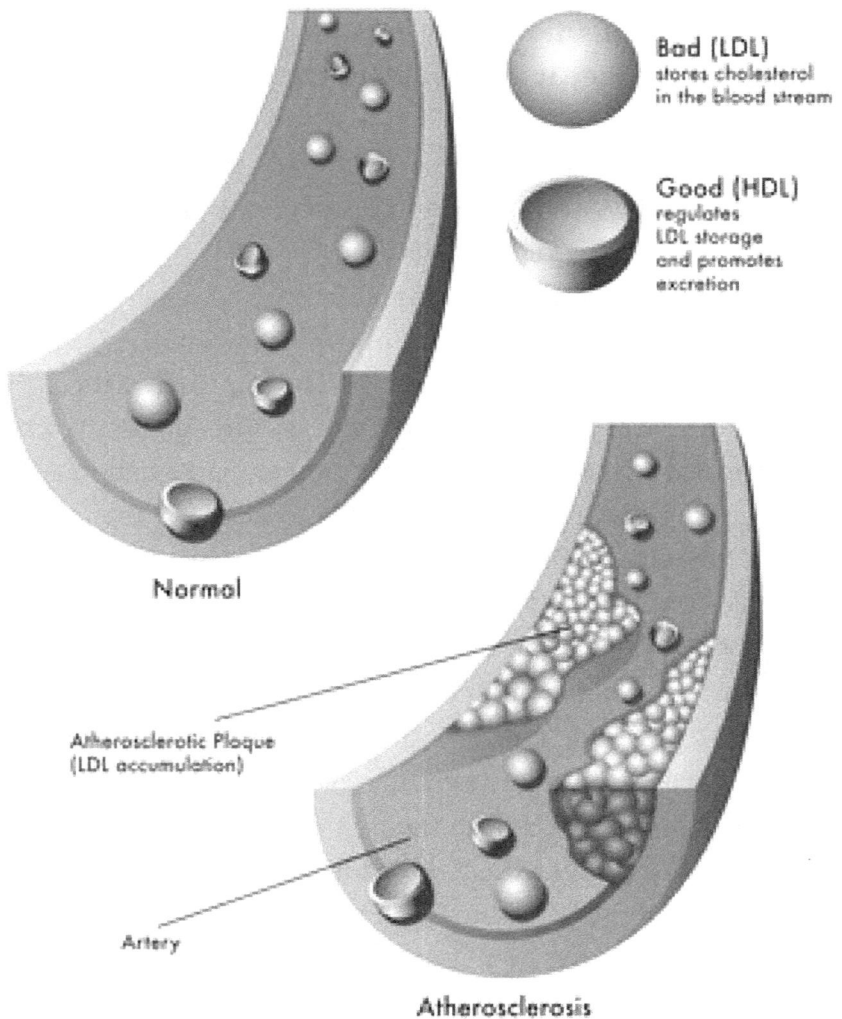

Bad (LDL)
stores cholesterol in the blood stream

Good (HDL)
regulates LDL storage and promotes excretion

Normal

Atherosclerotic Plaque (LDL accumulation)

Artery

Atherosclerosis

(© rob3000 - Fotolia.com)

Illustration of cholesterol in the bloodstream. Cholesterol is an essential ingredient. Without it, the body simply cannot survive.

The level of cholesterol is influenced by the fatty acids that enter the body via our food. Fatty acids as well are indispensable for the structure and functioning of the brain. We have to be careful with the amount of saturated fatty acids we ingest since they may elevate the cholesterol level in an undesired way.

Products that contain saturated fatty acids are among other things animal fats and oils, palm oil, coconut oil, sunflower oil, corn oil, and soy oil.

Unsaturated fatty acids, like omega-3 fatty acid, are very welcome because they play an important part in the communication between brain cells. They are also critical components of neuronal cell membranes. Omega-3 fatty acids have impressive anti-inflammatory power. Fatty fish like herring, mackerel, sardines, salmon, and anchovy are important sources, just like walnuts.

Deficits of unsaturated fatty acids are common in the aged brain. A deficiency of omega-3 fatty acids deteriorates communication between neurones and can lead to a diminished ability to concentrate and to forgetfulness. There even may exist a link between omega-3 fatty acids deficiency and dementia, as research in the US showed. Blood samples of a group of elderly were tested for fatty acids. Those participants who were accustomed to eat a lot of trans-fatty acids scored badly on memory tests and cognition tests. The effects of trans-fatty acids can be compared to those of saturated fatty acids. They abound in vegetable oils. Fried foods are rich in trans-fatty acids, as are for instance cakes and cookies since the baked goods industry uses a lot of partially hydrogenated oils which contain trans-fatty acids. Participants in the investigation, whose blood samples contained a lot of vitamin B, C, D, E, and omega-3 fatty acids, had the highest scores on the memory and cognition tests. When the researchers scanned the brains of these participants it became clear they also had a larger brain capacity than the participants who ingested a lot of trans-fatty acids.

Plaques

Just like any other cell in our body, our brain cells are directly affected by what we eat. That's why a lot of research has been done into possible links between certain nutrients and dementia.

One of the characteristics of dementia, as mentioned earlier, is the formation of minuscule plaques, clots of waste from brain metabolism, within the brain. These plaques hamper a smooth flow of information. This leads from one problem to another in the functioning of the brain. Many attention and effort in Alzheimer disease research is put into investigating ways to get rid of these plaques. According to several studies, red wine would counter the formation of these protein plaques and possibly even dissolve existing plaques. The same might be true for caffeine, present not only in coffee but also for instance in green tea.

Caffeine stimulates the brain by blocking chemicals that normally inhibit or slow neuronal activity. Physically, it can cause sweating, talkativeness, tinnitus, and hand tremors. Psychologically, it suppresses fatigue or drowsiness and increases feelings of alertness. One to three cups of coffee a day can improve work performance. Higher doses can produce agitation, headaches, nervousness, and a decreased ability to concentrate.

The incidence of Alzheimer disease is extremely low in India.

Scientists began to investigate what could be the cause of this. A very likely possibility is the spice curcuma, the substance that gives curry its yellow colour. The Indian cuisine is known for its extensive use of curcuma and curry. The spice also has a long history of use in Asian traditional medicines. Research is ongoing, but curcuma has been found to clearly have a positive effect on the clearance of protein plaques.

Researchers in the US looked at the influence of fish on the brain. They made brain scans of several hundred healthy people. Ten years later, they again scanned the brains of the same people. The participants who ate fish at least once a week turned out to have healthier brains than those who only ate fish from time to time or didn't eat it at all. Especially the brain parts susceptible to Alzheimer disease, like the hippocampus, were spared more extensively.

The study showed, if you eat fish at least once a week your risk of dementia diminishes. We're talking about baked or cooked fish here. Fried fish didn't turn out to contribute to a healthier brain.

It is not uncommon to see malnutrition among elderly people. This results in vitamin and mineral deficiencies, intensified by the fact that our bodies become less efficient at absorbing dietary nutrients as we age. Such deficiencies directly influence cognitive functioning.

Guideline

So just by eating the right way we can prevent problems in the ageing brain. Long-term habits of healthy eating have a positive effect on our cognitive functions. Diets rich in antioxidants and anti-inflammatory components, such as those in fruits, nuts, vegetables, and spices, may lower age-related cognitive decline and the risk of developing neurodegenerative diseases.

A study in Sweden confirmed it is not the effect of a single 'wonder' food on the body system that counts, but the power of multiple foods that makes the difference. A group of healthy, overweight people between 50 and 75 years of age were put on a diet of healthy foods for four weeks. After this period, the markers of inflammation in their body had reduced considerably and their memory and cognitive functions had improved.

If you want to get it right into the last detail you can use the following list as a guideline to put together your ideal menu. The list is based on the dietary advice of Andrew Weil, a well-known American doctor who tries to seduce people into a healthy lifestyle instead of relying solely on conventional medicine.

Vegetables and fruits are the basis for your healthy menu.

- Vegetables: 4-5 servings per day minimum (one serving is equal to 2 cups salad greens, ½ cup vegetables cooked, raw or juiced). Dark leafy greens, such as spinach, collard greens, kale, and Swiss chard are very healthy. This applies as well to cruciferous vegetables, such as broccoli, cabbage, Brussels sprouts, pak choi, and cauliflower. Other winners are carrots, beets, onions, peas, squashes, sea vegetables, and salad greens.

- Fruits: 3-4 servings per day (one serving is equal to 1 medium size piece of fruit, ½ cup chopped fruit, ¼ cup of dried fruit). Very good examples are raspberries, blueberries, strawberries, peaches, nectarines, oranges, pink grapefruit, red grapes, plums, pomegranates, blackberries, cherries, apples, and pears.

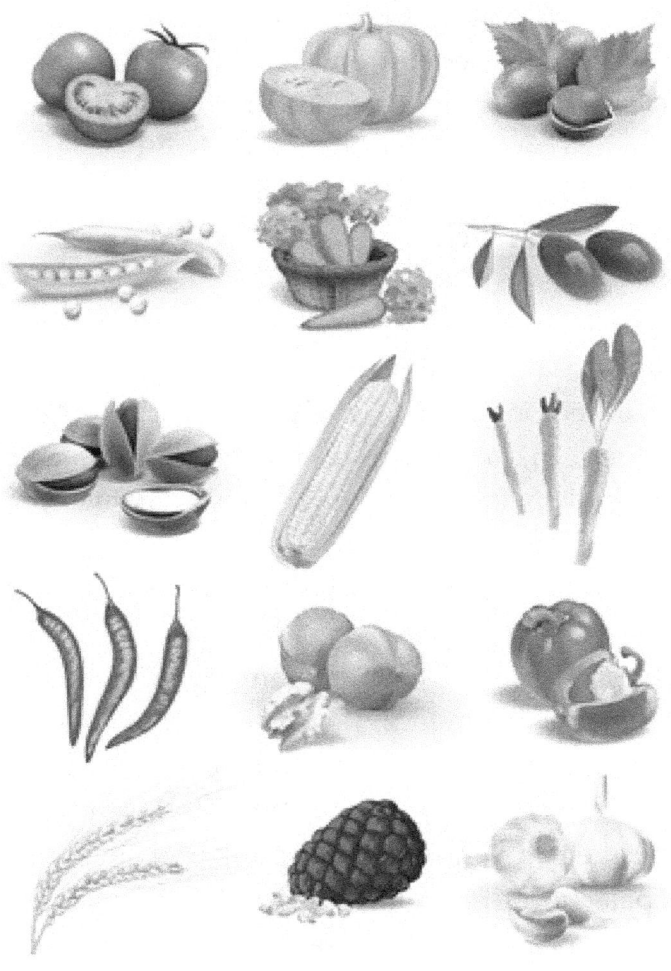

(© master24 – Fotolia.com)

By eating right, we can prevent problems in our ageing brain. Make your diet rich in antioxidants and anti-inflammatory components.

- Beans and legumes: 1-2 servings per day (one serving is equal to ½ cup cooked beans or legumes), for instance Anasazi, adzuki and black, beans as well as chickpeas, black-eyed peas, and lentils.

- Pasta: 2-3 servings per week (one serving is equal to about ½ cup cooked pasta), such as organic pasta, rice noodles, bean thread noodles, and part whole wheat and buckwheat noodles like Japanese udon and soba.

- Whole and cracked grains: 3-5 servings a day (one serving is equal to about ½ cup cooked grains). Healthy choices are brown rice, basmati rice, wild rice, buckwheat, groats, barley, quinoa, and steel-cut oats.

- Fats: 5-7 servings per day (one serving is equal to 1 teaspoon of oil, 2 walnuts, 1 tablespoon of flaxseed, 1 ounce of avocado). Healthy fats are extra virgin olive oil and expeller-pressed organic canola oil. Other sources of healthy fats include nuts (especially walnuts), avocados, and seeds, such as hemp seeds and freshly ground flaxseed.

- Fish and seafood: 2-6 servings per week (one serving is equal to 4 ounces of fish or seafood). The best choices are wild Alaskan salmon, herring, sardines, and black cod.

- Whole soy foods: 1-2 servings per day (one serving is equal to ½ cup tofu or tempeh, 1 cup soy milk, ½ cup cooked edamame, 1 ounce of soy nuts), preferably tofu, tempeh, edamame, soy nuts, and soy milk.

- Cooked Asian mushrooms: unlimited amounts. Healthy choices are shiitake, enokidake, maitake, oyster mushrooms.

- Other sources of protein: 1-2 servings a week (one portion is equal to 1 ounce of cheese, 1 eight-ounce serving of dairy, 1 egg, 3 ounces cooked poultry or skinless meat). Your best options are natural cheese and yogurt, omega-3 enriched eggs, skinless poultry, and grass-fed lean meats.

- Herbs and spices: unlimited amounts. Healthy choices are turmeric, curry powder, ginger, garlic, chilli peppers, basil, cinnamon, rosemary, and thyme.

- Drink water throughout the day, 2-4 cups of tea per day, preferably white, green, and oolong teas, and 1-2 glasses of red wine per day.

- Complete your healthy food trolley with a sound sweet every now and then. Examples are unsweetened dried fruit, dark chocolate, and fruit sorbet.

I can imagine, reading this extensive list, your head is spinning. It's quite a lot of food you have to deal with in one day. If you really want to stick to this guideline in every detail you will spend a lot of time every day shopping for groceries and preparing your meals. For most people, this complete package simply isn't feasible.

But that doesn't mean you have to drop out. Just start on the right foot with a few items on the list. You can certainly find some food stuffs you already have on your menu, which you enjoy eating and which are easy to prepare.

At the same time, strike some of the unhealthy products from your diet. From time to time, add one or two of the other items from the guideline to your menu. Thus, your menu will get healthier step by step.

11. BRAIN AEROBICS

New challenges put your brain on edge

Just after the Second World War the British Broadcasting Corporation introduced a radio program called Round Britain Quiz. This show is the oldest quiz still broadcast on British radio. Teams from various regions around the UK have to solve puzzles to be able to answer the quiz questions. Similar game shows have long been broadcasted on the US television channels. In 1938, Spelling Bee was the first television quiz program and Jeopardy! is one of the longest running and most popular game shows.

The broadcasting organisations were way ahead of their time. When they decided to introduce quiz programs on radio and television not much was known about the brain. Nowadays, more and more scientific evidence is emerging that quizzes and puzzles, in fact any kind of brain training, are very beneficial to your brain.

Among neuroscientists this fact is coined "use it or lose it", in other words: make sure you put your brain cells to work otherwise they will literally bore themselves to death. The brain is a flexible organ designed to improve with use. Due to the slow course of ageing in humans, the nervous system can compensate and maintain an adequate function even in centenarians.

Armed with this insight, more and more computer games and programs are spilled onto the market directed at training the brain. Quite a lot of companies try to get a piece of the cake, capitalising on the growing attention for and fear of dementia. The sales pitches are promising. Those who give way to the brain games will be awarded with a better memory, enhanced creativity, more efficient and faster data processing in the brain, faster reflexes, enhanced concentration, and improved multi-tasking, in short, will develop a more clever brain. Devoting ten minutes a day to such a brain game is all that is necessary to end up with a fitter brain, claim the ads.

And so we go to the shop and diligently buy a computer, this time not for the (grand) children, but for ourselves. Or we subscribe to some website supplying games for the brain. In the long run, many of those games are not really captivating. Besides, they have a rather competitive edge while we on the other hand are in a more relaxed phase of life in which we don't find it very necessary anymore to constantly aim for a higher score. Those games even sometimes have a slight addictive effect. You experience a kind of pressing obligation to obediently do your portion of games every day. The culmination of mockery is a game that determines the age of your brain. It is quite a feat the computer can decide, after you have done a few puzzles, the age of your brain is 33 while you have long passed the age of 60…

Stimulate

It seems that the brain needs mental challenges to retain its functionality. Just as physical fitness is improved by exercising the body the hypothesis is that cognitive abilities can be maintained or improved by exercising the brain. Scientific support for this hypothesis is still limited. Some evidence exists that high levels of mental activity are associated with reduced risk of age-related dementia.

The influence of mental activity on the brain has to do with neurogenesis, the birth of new neurones. In rats, it has been shown novel environments trigger neurogenesis. They get more new neurones when they live in cages with interesting toys.

To be able to explore this fascinating, new environment the rats need to use their brains intensively. They need new neurones to be able to get to know the new things and find new routes and to store this information in their memories. The brains of rats living in the same, dull environment all the time don't need neurogenesis. Everything is known and the animal can function with the knowledge it has, stored in the existing neurones.

In humans, the birth of new brain cells and the effect mental activity has on them have also been studied. Preliminary results show mental exercise may increase the rate at which new brain cells survive and make functional connections into existing neural networks.

It so happens, a large part of the new-born neurones won't survive. Their survival depends on activity. Only stimulated neurones survive and make it into adulthood.

When certain parts of the brain are activated the glia cells and neurones in that area release various chemicals. These chemicals activate the new neurones and make sure they will develop and start making contacts with other neurones.

Thus, only when the brain is confronted with something new, new neurones will be recruited.

This way, the rats in the laboratory raised in enriched environments learn better and have a better memory than their colleagues in the empty cages. Thanks to the extra neurones, their brain weight is about 5 percent higher in the cerebral cortex as a whole and 9 percent higher in the stimulated areas, such as the hippocampus.

An additional advantage is that stimulating your brain possibly has a positive effect on the amount of REM sleep you experience at night. REM sleep is the active form of sleep, which we need among other things to store memories. Babies spend half of their total sleeping time in REM sleep. In older people, REM sleep constitutes only fifteen to twenty percent of their total sleeping time. This may have to do with the fact that babies learn many new things that have to be recorded in memory.

Many elderly people suffer memory problems. Their limited amount of REM sleep may be involved in this. New experiences, learning new knowledge and skills, and training the brain may also enhance the time spent in REM sleep in adults and thus boost memory functioning. This important research path still needs further investigation.

In shape

When you challenge and engage your brain, especially by learning new skills, it probably will be healthier and function better. A trained brain stays in shape. The brain has to be stimulated during its whole lifetime. To do something new or learn something gives rise to new connections between neurones. The more of these connections exist, the better it is. If in the course of time some connections are lost due to for instance disease, a concussion or toxic substances you will still have enough connections left. The brain finds alternative neural routes to be able to fulfil as much of its functions as possible.

Research shows ever more clearly your personal way of living has an enormous influence on how your brain is functioning. This applies to people who live at present, in our current societies. Of course, numerous examples exist of grandfathers and grandmothers who reached very high ages possessing full mental powers, but who lived in a - for us now - very unhealthy way. Maybe they drank heavily, they smoked their cigars or cigarettes, they only finished elementary school, and they undertook nothing to stimulate their brains.

But those grandfathers and grandmothers were born in completely different times than the ones we are living in. Not only will we all generally reach far higher ages than the people who were old say fifty years ago, but during our lifetime we are also exposed to much more unhealthy influences than they were. We move far less, we often eat unhealthier, and we suffer far more devastating stress, which causes our cells to age more rapidly and exhibit deficiencies.

An American scientist came up with an original way to find proof for the influence of lifestyle on cognitive functioning. In 1986, he started researching the link between ageing and brain diseases. This is nothing out of the ordinary, but the group of elderly he used for his research is unique. He found a group of 678 Roman Catholic sisters in the US willing to participate in the study that is ongoing even now. They were between 75 and 102 years of age when the study began and undergo annual assessments of their cognitive and physical function. They also donate their brains for research purposes after their deaths.

In itself a group of nuns isn't quite a good intersection of society. On the other hand, all the nuns do have a rather comparable way of living in the same kind of environment. Therefore, the study results are not influenced by differences in external circumstances, such as the use of alcohol or drugs, and giving birth. One of the results from the study so far is that nuns that lead intellectually challenging lives show more moderate declines in intellectual skills when ageing. Most of the participating nuns have jobs in education and generally keep on working until very high age. The nuns that keep active this way are clearly better off than their colleagues who owing to certain circumstances experience a more quiet old age.

Reserve

So it appears useful after retirement to pass on your knowledge in one way or the other, not only for the young people who would benefit from your know-how and experience, but also for yourself because of the positive effect this has on the functioning of your own brain.

Education in itself also seems to be beneficial for your brain. More years of education appear to be linked to less age-related cognitive decline. This property has been labelled cognitive reserve, representing the brain's resilience to damage. A higher reserve may mean established networks in the brain are more efficient, have a greater capacity, and are less susceptible to disruption. It also allows the brain to compensate through alternative networks in the presence of declines by ageing or disease.

Of course this information won't do you much good when you have finished your formal education many years ago, apart from the fact that you could impress the utmost importance of continued education on your children and grandchildren. But there is still hope. Not only education in your younger years contributes to the reserve capacity of your brain, but also interesting activities you have undertaken as an adult, and even for instance the language course you are attending at later age.

A comment is certainly in order as far as this theory about education and cognitive reserve is concerned. Studies have shown a role of education in age-related cognitive decline in the western world. In other parts of the world though, this link has not been confirmed. India and West-Africa for instance have the lowest prevalence rates of Alzheimer disease among the elderly despite a lack of formal schooling or literacy training. Apart from cognitive reserve, other factors, such as cultural, racial, and economic influences, surely also play a role in cognitive decline.

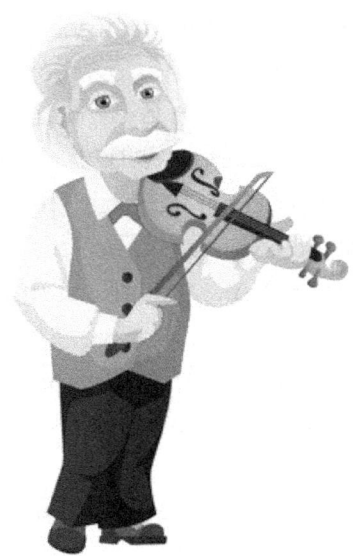

(© RA Studio - Fotolia.com)

Physicist Albert Einstein played the violin to activate different parts of his brain and thus bolster his creativity.

It is a fact that as we age, we hardly do any intensive learning anymore. In middle age, most people are replaying skills mastered a long time ago. This means that in old age the systems that keep the brain flexible and are involved in setting up new networks may have not been engaged for over forty years.

Therefore it is so important to keep an open mind and be susceptible to new influences. To learn something new or do something that requires your full attention will keep your brain flexible. The world-renowned physicist Albert Einstein played the violin to activate other parts of his brain and thus bolster his creativity. British politician Winston Churchill did the same by painting landscapes.

Juggle

Learning new skills is an excellent way to stimulate the brain's plastic abilities. An interesting experiment was done at the University of Jena in Germany. A group of healthy senior citizens, mean age 60 years, and a group of 20-year old adolescents were trained for a period of three months to juggle with three balls. Having completed the training, the elderly were clearly less proficient than the younger participants. Only 23 percent of the older group learned to keep the three balls in the air for sixty seconds, whereas 100 percent of the younger group succeeded in doing this.

But most surprisingly, both groups showed the same plasticity in the same brain regions when their brains were scanned. In both groups, increases in grey matter occurred in the brain regions necessary for the juggling skill. These changes were transient. After interruption of the practice, the increases gradually disappeared.

The experiment shows there is absolutely no doubt, learning a new skill can bring about changes and create new networks also in an aged brain. To achieve this you don't even have to really master the new skill.

Of several other activities we now also know what changes they produce in the brain. People who are bilingual have more neurones and more connections in a part of the left hemisphere dedicated to language. Learning a new language at later age has a similar, but less intense influence.

The hippocampus, mentioned several times already, is important in spatial skills. Animals appear to have a larger hippocampus when they need more spatial skills. Monogamous pine voles for instance have a smaller hippocampus than polygamous meadow voles, especially where the males are concerned. The last species occupies larger range sizes to find females.

A study of the brains of cab drivers in London showed they too have a significantly larger hippocampus than other people. To get the job as taxi driver, they have to pass a difficult exam and show an extensive knowledge of the street plan of Britain's capital.

The more years a taxi driver is on the job, the more complex routes and locations he memorises. A more experienced taxi driver thus has a larger hippocampus than his colleague who has just started.

The frequent use of GPS navigation devices seems to shrink our hippocampus.

Music

Two activities clearly stand out as far as their positive influence on the brain is concerned: dancing and making music. Both activities use a large number of different parts in the brain since they combine movement and cognition.

It is not only great fun and entertaining to go to dance classes, but also very beneficial to your brain for three reasons. One, you get to know new people and make new contacts. Two, acquiring the dance steps is a mental challenge. Three, dancing is an excellent form of exercise that also requires balance and coordination.

Researchers in Canada chose the tango as best type of dance for elderly people. The fancy footwork required to perform the tango bolsters brainpower. Dancing the tango also improves balance since you have to move within a restricted area without losing your footing.

For the study, researchers recruited 30 seniors aged 62 to 90. Half the group was assigned to a tango lessons group and the other half to a walking group. After ten weeks, the tango group showed more improvement in balance, posture and motor coordination, as well as cognitive gains, than the walking group.

Scientists have done rather a lot of looking around in the brains of musicians. They came up with intriguing conclusions.

Making music in general engages large parts of the brain. Playing an instrument combines visual, motor, and auditory skills and memory. Musicians have more neurones in the brain regions involved in these skills. These effects increase with the duration and the intensity of their training.

The physical ability to play an instrument also generates changes in the brain. In violin players for instance, more area in their motor cortex is devoted to pathways representing the thumb and fifth finger of their left hand. The younger they begin practicing, the larger this area is. In the brains of musicians who play other instruments, areas for other fingers are enlarged.

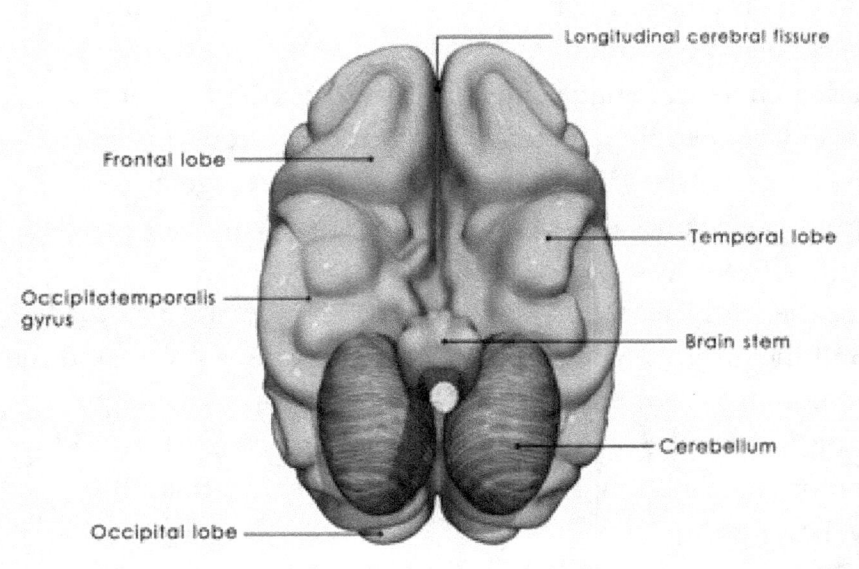

Longitudinal cerebral fissure

Frontal lobe

Temporal lobe

Occipitotemporalis gyrus

Brain stem

Cerebellum

Occipital lobe

The cerebellum plays an important role in coordinating movement. Musicians have a larger cerebellum than people who don't make music.

Musicians have a larger cerebellum, Latin for little brain, which is attached to the bottom of the brain underneath the cerebral hemispheres. This region of the brain plays an important role in coordinating movement. Alcohol readily affects the cerebellum, hence the uncontrolled movements of someone who is drunk. Out of this motor control function, the cerebellum most probably also is crucial to timing in making music.

In order to perform bimanual complex motor sequences – and for some instruments both feet are involved as well -, musicians need an increased and fast cooperation between both cerebral hemispheres. This results in an enlarged corpus callosum, the bundle of neural fibres that connects the left and the right hemisphere and facilitates inter-hemispheric communication.

The beauty of all this is of course that all this extra brain capacity not only is available for making music, but can be used for other activities as well. Whether musicians suffer dementia less frequently thanks to their reserve capacity is difficult to study. Many musicians die long before they could have been stricken with dementia due to other causes such as alcohol, drugs, performing in smoky environments, and an unhealthy style of living. But it is a fact that among musicians who do reach old age, very few cases of dementia are known.

Chat

To socialise with other people also plays a role in preventing cognitive decline. What's, more, social isolation can bring about mental decline. Various studies among many thousands of elderly have shown social involvement and maintaining relationships with other people help protect mental powers against ageing.

Why that is so, is not clear yet. Maybe it is because associating socially constitutes a challenge and thus stimulates neural networks. When you live a socially active life you have to remember a lot of things of many different people through which you make use of your memory more frequently. Furthermore, your brain networks will be activated when you keep an open mind towards other people and try to understand other people's ideas and opinions.

Less frequent participation in social activities is even associated with a more rapid decline in motor function, researchers in the US concluded. They annually assessed a group of almost one thousand older individuals for a period of five years, looking at basic motor function, including muscle strength in the arms and legs, and motor performance, including walking and balance. Motor function decline was more rapid in those who less frequently participated in social activities. This may have to do with the fact that human social interaction is very complex. Many parts of the brain are involved, among which the networks that combine input for planning and executing certain behaviour. Those same networks also take part in planning and executing certain movements. Possibly, stimulating those networks for one task also produces a positive effect on the other task.

The fact that chances of an extensive social life generally decrease when you grow older constitutes a major problem. You will retire and lose contacts you had via your job, your children live far away, and your circle of friends becomes smaller since some friends die before you. In those circumstances, the thing to do is to look for other social activities, for example via clubs, courses, or volunteer work. But also a chat with the mailman, with the shop assistant or with the waitress in the coffee shop would cater for your needs.

A supportive social network has a protective effect on cognitive performance. People simply do better if they get out of their houses and interact with others.

Games

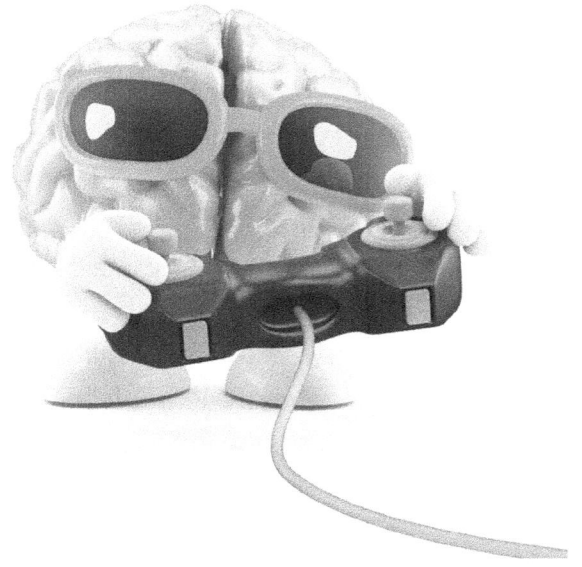

(© Steve Young – Fotolia.com)

Playing computer games does not boost mental skills in general, but you will get better at the specific tasks trained via a game.

And what about those computer games? That's a question everyone would like to get answered, above all of course the manufacturers of computer games. The effects of computer games on the brain can be measured in different ways. The most trustworthy scientific investigations consist of a brain scan of the participants before and after the brain training to see what kind of differences it has produced. Such an investigation requires a lot of money. That's why most researchers use tests. The participants in a study take a test before and after the brain training. If the tests results are better the second time, the training was a success.

So far, studies of the effect of brain training haven't come up with unambiguous results. From most studies, the conclusion can be drawn participants are getting better at the tasks that have been trained via the computer game. In the UK, over 11,000 volunteers between 18 and 60 years of age took part in an online training program. After a total of at least 4 hours training, the participants had improved in the specific trained tasks, but there was no improvement on tests measuring general cognitive abilities. A cognitive training intervention with 2800 participants between 65 and 94 years of age in the US came up with the same result. Reliable signs of improvement were shown on the targeted cognitive abilities, but no training effects were measured on everyday functioning.

Neurobics, as brain training sometimes is called, does not boost mental skills in general. You don't end up with a more clever and fit brain.

Exceptions are training programs for the brain based on the conclusions of scientific research. Normal ageing comes with progressive functional losses in perception, cognition, and memory. As the brain keeps its capacity for plasticity and adaptive reorganisation during its lifetime, an appropriately designed training program should be able to counteract this decline.

A few neuroscientists have stepped into this specialty. They make use of the neuroplasticity of our brain. Plasticity exists from cradle to grave and improvements in cognitive functioning are possible in the elderly as well. Even the aged brain is flexible enough to shift tasks to other networks. The brain is perfectly capable of finding an alternative route if one route for the transfer of information is blocked.

The scientifically based training programs incite the brain to bring this flexibility into action to perform tasks that have become more difficult due to ageing. The programs contain exercises for audition and vision. Training these two parts of the sensory system turns out to have positive effects on the speed of data processing and on the ability to concentrate and to remember.

A large group of healthy seniors in the US took part in a study to test one of those scientifically based brain training programs. After finishing the training, no less than 87 percent of the participants showed considerable improvement in their cognitive skills. They were better at recognition and discrimination and scored higher on memory tests. The enhancement was sustained five years later, even without additional training.

The American neuroscientist Michael Merzenich, one of the developers of such a scientifically based brain training program and a firm believer in the beneficial effects of brain training focused on neuroplasticity, puts it like this: "Brain exercises may be as useful as drugs to treat diseases as severe as schizophrenia."

12. THE MOVING BRAIN

Physical exercise keeps your brain healthy

Two thousand years ago, the Romans already hit the nail right on the head when the poet Juvenal declared: mens sana en corpore sano – a healthy mind in a healthy body. By now, we all know very well we have to keep moving to stay healthy. Information campaigns about the importance of exercise for heart health and the condition of blood vessels have done their job.

But it is not only indispensable to stay in shape and for supple muscles that we have to engage in some form of physical exercise, it is also imperative for the brain. Weird as it may seem, regular movement may be the single most important activity you absolutely cannot skip if you want to keep your brain healthy.

In fact, we developed a brain in the first place to be able to move. During evolution, our brains got better and better in getting our bodies to move in the most adequate manner. Adequate movements, like running away when an enemy comes too close or being able to pluck that small berry from its branch with our fingers and to put it into our mouth, are after all indispensable for our survival.

Only organisms that move from place to place appear to need a brain, as far as we now know. A very special case is that of the sea squirt. Many sea squirts swim about like a tadpole when they are young. They have a brain and a nerve cord. As adults, they attach themselves permanently to a rock and become sedentary. They gradually absorb and digest their brain and nerve cord.

The animals don't move anymore and evidently no longer need their brain and nerve cord. What's more, the brain cannot handle the fact that the body of the animal isn't moving anymore and dies. Stronger evidence for the utmost importance of moving would be hard to find.

Movement

The human brain is also directed at movement. The brain as it exists now came into being about 100,000 years ago as a result of parts being added or adapted during evolution. During all this time, movement has been the most important activity of human beings. Movement while hunting for food for your own survival and movement while procreating to make sure your genes are going to survive. Cognition, the process of thinking and reasoning, came into play much, much later. That's why our brain still is mainly adjusted to movement. And that is where modern man has gone wrong. Thanks to the way he has organised societies he is undertaking less and less physical activity. Hence the malfunctioning body system and the diseases. When a brain is starting to decline in old age, cognition is the first function to be affected. The motor functions of the brain remain in good condition far longer. Simultaneously

The human body is designed for regular and varied use. We cannot survive without movement. Physical activity needs the brain, namely the motor function. But conversely physical activity is just as vital to every other brain function, including memory, emotion, and language.

Movement is also a major player in learning. In infants,

development of motor functions such as crawling, standing, and walking, influences their reading and writing skills and also their visual development. Through a series of studies, researchers in the Netherlands have been able to establish physical exercise has a very positive effect on the learning performance of students between six and eighteen years of age.

Our cognitive functions have evolved from movement and still depend on it. A lot of brain function is essentially movement. Movement is inseparably tied to cognition. It is not by chance the part of the brain where movements are coordinated, the motor cortex, is located in the frontal lobes, where executive functions are performed.

The frontal lobes process motor and mental functions simultaneously. This parallel handling helps to master a skill, such as driving a car, for which you not only have to act, but also have to think. The interaction between neural networks for movement and for cognition turns out to be extremely useful. This is why you sometimes suddenly come up with the solution to a problem while taking a walk, even while you were not consciously thinking about the problem.

Another part of the brain is an important player in both movement and cognition as well. The cerebellum, located at the bottom of the brain in the back, coordinates physical movement, but also the thinking process, which is after all a kind of mental movement. It is responsible for balance, posture, precision, and coordination, but is also involved – as has been discovered only recently - in cognitive functions such as shifting attention, planning, and verbal working memory.

Message

Chemically, a lot is going on in your brain during exercise. To be able to move there's a need for the neurotransmitter acetylcholine. This chemical substance, made by neurones, makes sure information from the brain gets to the muscles. If for a certain movement a muscle in your leg has to contract, the order to do so comes from the motor cortex in your brain. Acetylcholine activates one neurone after another in the network until the message finally has reached the muscle.

This neurotransmitter isn't only involved in information transfer from the brain to the muscles and back. It is also involved in complex mental processes such as learning, memory, sleeping, and dreaming. Besides, it influences alertness and attention.

When you are exercising, production of acetylcholine is increased to make sure all the necessary movements can be executed in the right way. Increased levels of the neurotransmitter result in increased arousal and wakefulness. That's why you feel really awake after exercising.

At the same time, the extra quantity of acetylcholine may also have a positive effect on learning and memory, not only in a direct way but also indirectly.

This neurotransmitter triggers longer periods of REM sleep. And we already have learned REM sleep is extremely important for learning and memory.

Exercise also increases levels of other neurotransmitters like dopamine and serotonin. These neurotransmitters help regulate mood and control anxiety. They make you feel relaxed and able to handle stress and aggression.

That's why regular exercise is such an effective medicine against depression, the most frequently occurring emotional disorder among elderly. Exercise has been shown to reduce depression and prevent its recurrence.

Researchers in the US followed nearly fifty thousand women for ten years. The women who reported exercising most were less likely to be diagnosed as depressed. At the same time, the time the women spent watching television turned out to be of influence on their chance of getting depressed. The more hours per week in front of the screen, the higher the risk of depression. The researchers concluded you have to limit the time watching television and increase the time spent exercising to reduce your chance of depression.

Robust physical exercise may be as effective as medication in treating depression, without the negative side effects of pharmaceuticals. Exercise activates the release of endorphins that create an overall feeling of well-being; it regulates body rhythms; it improves self-esteem; and it provides social support. The only problem is that for depressed people it is difficult to find the energy and the motivation to begin an exercise regime.

Vulnerable

Our great friend, the hippocampus, is also very fond of physical exercise. Exercise has been shown to increase neurogenesis, the birth of new neurones, in the hippocampus. These new neurones most probably are indispensable for learning and memorising new facts. Several factors may contribute to the fact that neurogenesis diminishes, such as long-term stress, poor sleep, and the ageing process. The hippocampus is very exposed to ageing. Anything to lend the vulnerable hippocampus a helping hand is welcome of course.

Experiments with mice in a laboratory have shown physical exercise indeed counteracts the decline in neurogenesis. Aged mice that had been sedentary were given the possibility to enter a running wheel. Voluntarily, they ran their daily training rounds in the wheel.

Apparently, mice know better what's good for them than we do. Neither are they being distracted by other temptations like watching television.

After one month of running, the aged mice showed faster acquisition and better retention of a water maze than age-matched controls that didn't run. The number of new neurones in their hippocampus proved to have risen dramatically.

This shows it is possible to thwart the decline in neurogenesis and the shrinking of the hippocampus at later age by exercising. Elderly people in good physical shape turn out to have a larger hippocampus than their contemporaries who don't exercise. And a healthy, sizeable hippocampus offers protection against dementia.

In the previous chapter, we already saw intellectual stimulation or living in an enriched environment has the same positive effect on neurogenesis. When comparing the effects of physical and mental exercise, in a very broad sense it seems physical exercise creates new neurones and stimulates their proliferation while learning enhances the survival of these neurones and their incorporation into existing neural networks.

Therefore, it is not very useful to train your brain mentally without any form of physical training. The perfect combination is regular exercise and learning or undertaking something new from time to time.

Oxygen

When we grow older, the blood flow to the brain diminishes. One of the reasons for this process is the fact that walls of the blood vessels harden. Less oxygen reaches the brain and this starts a chain reaction of problems. The brain depends on oxygen for its survival. The cortex, the folded outer layer of the brain, and again the hippocampus are particularly vulnerable to oxygen deprivation.

Mental processes in the elderly have been shown to improve when extra oxygen is administered. But don't go running to an oxygen bar to inhale a dose of oxygen. It is bad for the lungs to receive a lot of oxygen in this artificial way. Besides, other nasty side effects may occur, for example when the equipment hasn't been cleaned sufficiently.

It is not at all necessary to reach for extra oxygen in such a drastic manner. Physical activity augments the number and density of blood vessels. It brings about an increase in the cerebral blood flow and thus a better oxygenation. Besides, it lowers your heartbeat and blood pressure. These are very positive facts for your brain as well.

Glucose

Exercise also helps the cells absorb glucose. The glucose our body extracts from the food we eat, stimulates the pancreas to make insulin.

As discussed before, neurones need insulin to be able to take up this glucose, which is their main energy source.

Insulin is like the valve of a fuel dispenser at a filling station through which gasoline flows into the fuel tank of your car. Successively, this gasoline will keep your motor running.

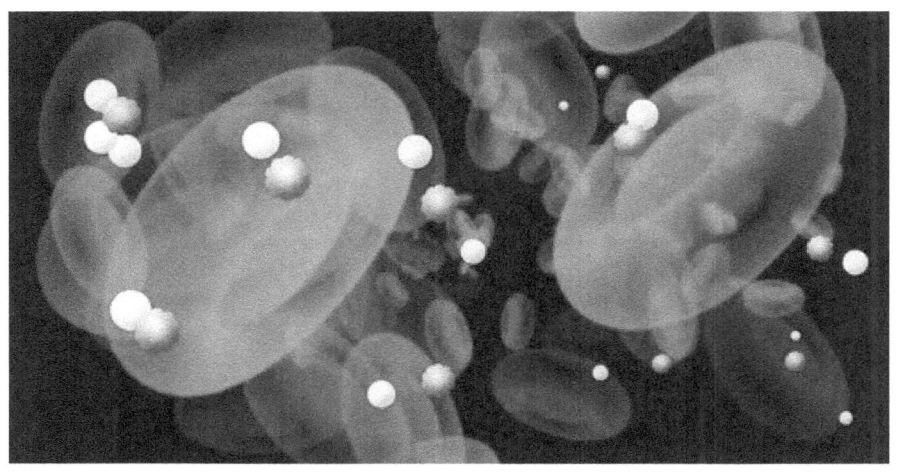

Image of the bloodstream showing red blood cells, glucose, and insulin. Exercise helps restore insulin sensitivity and thus improves absorption of glucose.

A greater difficulty handling glucose is part of the ageing process. Older cells aren't as sensitive to insulin anymore. It is as if the opening of the fuel tank is clogged up and the valve won't enter very well. Consequently, glucose can't enter into the neurones. The brain is inundated by unused fuel. This surplus of glucose makes the cells age more rapidly. Thus, the brain is more vulnerable to neurodegenerative diseases. Since the pancreas keeps on creating insulin, this also results in too high insulin levels. This may lead to type 2 diabetes. Many older adults suffer this type of diabetes. People with type 2 diabetes have chronically elevated levels of blood glucose. This excess of glucose is detrimental, among others to the cells in the hippocampus. As a consequence, people with type 2 diabetes are more susceptible to memory problems.

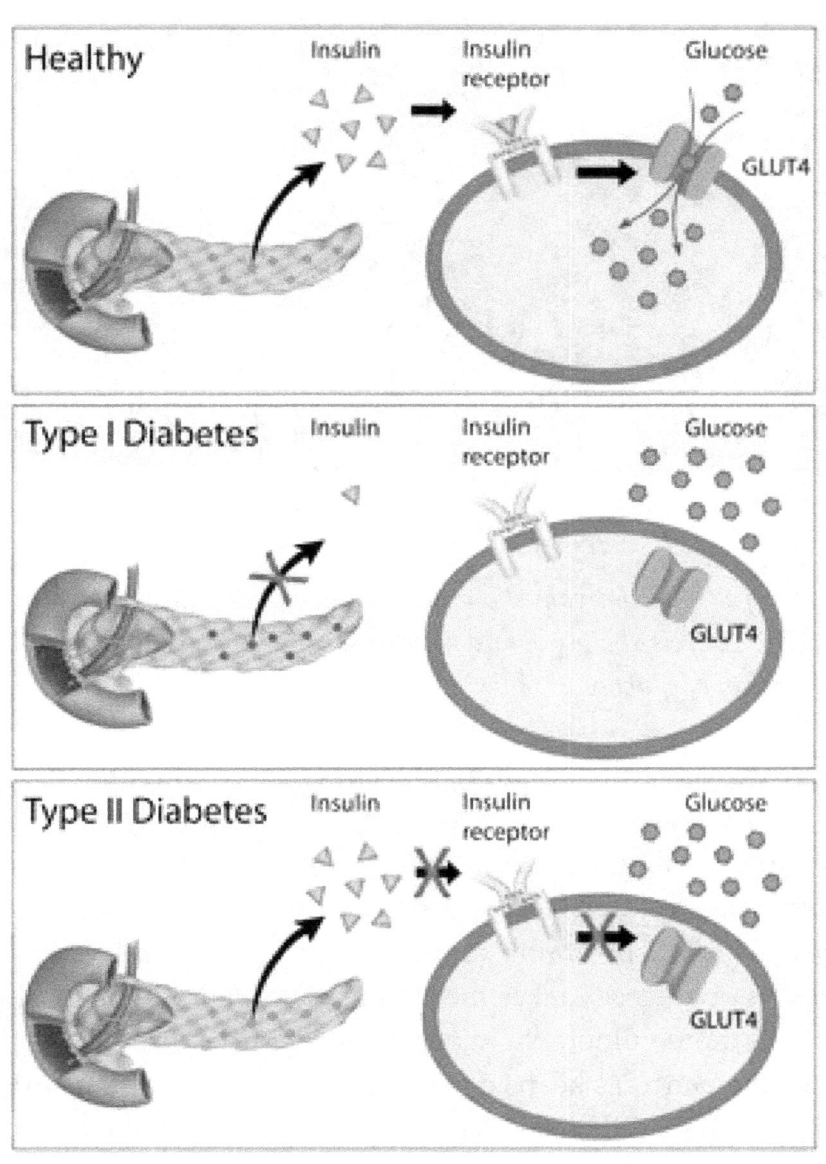

(© Alila Medical Media – Fotolia.com)

Insulin helps glucose enter a cell. The cell needs this glucose to keep its motor running. In a person who suffers diabetes, this process is disturbed.

Exercise helps restore insulin sensitivity and thus improves absorption of glucose. It is a simple and safe way to regulate blood glucose levels and to preserve the hippocampus and thus protect memory and cognitive functions.

We have all experienced it every now and then: such a wonderful, intense sleep after you have been outdoors for the day. Physical activities help combat insomnia. It makes you sleep longer and seemingly better as well.

Our sleeping pattern comprises several stages which you go through several times during the night. Exercise increases the time you spend in the deepest sleep stage. This is the restorative sleep during which your immune system is recharged.

Understandably, people who exercise regularly, have a better functioning immune system and are thus better equipped to stand up to influenza attacks. When they do catch a cold it usually is far less intense than in people who largely lead sedentary lives.

Mass

By far the most important established outcome is that exercise boosts brain power. It makes the brain function better. Several research studies have compared the brains of healthy elderly who exercise regularly with those of healthy elderly who hardly move. Exercising older adults perform better on cognitive tasks and they have clearly more brain mass than seniors who lead a more sedentary life. Training also enhances the plasticity of brain networks.

In one of the studies, elderly people participated in a walking program. They used a treadmill for forty minutes, three times a week. After one year, their neurones had grown many more connections and their neural networks had developed. This increased connectivity resulted in improvement in executive function. The participants had improved on planning, organisation, and coordination and their working memory functioned better. Exactly those tasks that become a bit more difficult with ageing. Logically, positive effects were also noticed on brain regions involved in coordinating movement. It took a while before improvements became noticeable and measurable. When the investigators tested the participants after six months of training, they found no significant effects yet. Those results only showed up after participants had trained for a year. So it is a matter of perseverance!

This was also clear from research into the effect of walking on possible memory problems at later age. Nearly three hundred people walked between six to nine miles a week for a period of nine years. Those who walked most had a larger brain mass than those who walked less distance. Besides, the top walkers cut the risk of developing memory problems in half. Walking at least six miles a week may protect brain size and thus preserve memory in old age.

Long-term exercise may even slow the onset or the progression of Alzheimer disease. In a study with special mice with Alzheimer disease, after five months of voluntary exercise in their running wheels the mice had considerably less senile plaques, clumps of insoluble protein between neurones that are one of the most characteristic physical signs of Alzheimer disease in the brain.

While mental training appears to promote positive changes in the brain and in processing speed, the only single method tested in people so far that has shown generalised improvement in brain function and capacity is exercise. It affects the most basic aspects of the brain's functional architecture. Physical activity moderates undesirable age-related changes in cognition, brain function, and brain structure. There's no doubt older people who continue to be active are best at resisting cognitive decline. In general, the more active older adults are the healthier and happier they are.

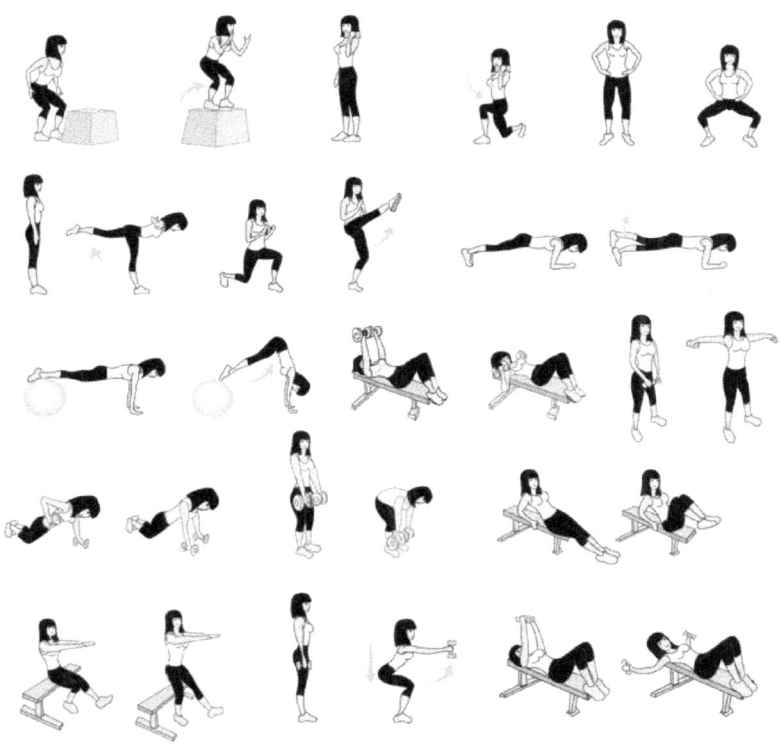

(© onanana - Fotolia.com)

Aerobic exercise generates a very positive health effect on the brain. The general guideline is at least 30 minutes, five times a week.

Endurance

Physical activity and exercise are rather extensive concepts. What kind of exercise and what amount would be necessary to keep your brain healthy?

Generally speaking, physical exercise is any bodily activity that enhances physical fitness, overall health, and wellness.

It comprises three segments:

- Aerobic exercise, such as walking, swimming, cycling, dancing, rope-skipping, and working out on exercise machines, focusses on increasing cardiovascular endurance. It is performed at moderate levels of intensity for an extended period of time.

- Anaerobic exercise, such as weight training and sprinting, increases short-term muscle strength. Sports like tennis, golf, football, basketball, and downhill skiing are also considered anaerobic exercise.

- Flexibility exercise, such as stretching and swinging, improves the range of motion of muscles and joints and is intended to make you more loose-limbed.

Aerobic exercise is what has been proven to generate a very positive health effect on the brain. It is not clear yet how much exercise you need to enjoy its benefits.

Overly vigorous exercising is not good as it releases excess free radicals and impairs the immune system. Top athletes as a rule don't live very long. Apparently, the enormous physical exertion required to play sports at top level shortens the human lifespan.

For the moment, the general guideline for beneficial exercise is at least 30 minutes, five times a week. It will take some time for the results to be noticed. Many of the positive actions for instance go on at cell level and you won't notice them, but in the long run they do make a difference for your brain health. By the way, it is useful to combine aerobic exercise with strength training and flexibility and balance training. Strength training helps to maintain bone and muscle mass. Flexibility and balance training is beneficial to reduce physical discomfort and to protect from falls.

The only minus among all this good news is that you have to keep on moving, for the rest of your life. Exercising has to be a continuing pursuit. You can't save up some extra health by exercising now and putting it to use later. Of course, the positive results of moving on your brain and body will be present for some time after you would have stopped exercising. Your health will be going downhill irrevocably though when you do not move enough anymore. Proper exercise will always remain just as important as a healthy diet. It should become a standard part of your way of life. But that shouldn't be too hard, now we know what terrific processes are going on in your brain while exercising. There is no greater reward than a healthy brain!

Excuses

Of course, we have all known for a long time we should move more often. It is necessary if you want to stay slim and for keeping heart and blood vessels healthy. Then why don't we do it? Why aren't we exercising enthusiastically, just like the aged mice, without thinking, simply because we instinctively know it is good for us? Why do we sometimes start with the best of intentions, but do we almost always give up again loaded with excuses for why we can't do our exercise today? Maybe it's exactly because we can think and reason. Because most of the times somewhere in our consciousness a little voice comes up that produces all kinds of important reasons why we have to do other things and thus naturally don't have any time left for exercise.

For most people, the knowledge that exercise is important to maintain and improve health isn't enough to encourage them to stop watching television for half an hour and get up out of their chairs. They apparently don't link their aches and pains with a sedentary lifestyle. Or they cannot bring themselves to suffer a bit before harvesting the benefits of a more trained body. And the long-term rewards of postponing age-related decline seem to be too far away.

The organisation of the brain itself is one of the obstacles for changing the way you live. As explained in the first part of this book, neurones have their fixed, favourite contacts. Beaten tracks between neurones are easier travelled. It is hard to get off those established pathways, to make new connections.

Routine

That's why we so often get stuck in routines, especially when we get older and mental flexibility declines. Routine is a good thing. It brings rest and regularity into daily activities and offers grip. But too many fixed habits are bad. They give you a very hard time to introduce adjustments into your lifestyle. On top of that, the neurotransmitter dopamine seems to play a role in plasticity. Neurotransmitters make sure information gets from one neurone to the next and dopamine does that among other things in the neural networks responsible for a change of behaviour. People with low dopamine levels have problems breaking out of routine. One of the brain parts where the neurotransmitter dopamine is produced is very sensitive to ageing. Because of this, less dopamine becomes available.

Dopamine is also the main transmitter in reward systems in the brain. When we do something we like, a lot of dopamine is released. This makes us feel good and come back for more. Sitting in front of the television and watching a funny sitcom for instance instead of going to the gym.

Endorphins also function as neurotransmitters in the reward systems. Whereas dopamine is involved in wanting a reward, endorphins are associated with the actual enjoyment of the reward. They suppress pain and increase the release of dopamine.

Endorphins are also released when eating chocolate, laughing, smiling, touching, meditating, singing, listening to music, having an orgasm, etcetera. They are associated with euphoric moods. Runner's high for instance is a condition in which the body is pushed beyond endurance and pain turns to pleasure due to the production of endorphins.

Fortunately, also during exercise extra dopamine is produced since this neurotransmitter is needed as well for coordinating movement. So, once we have forced ourselves to begin exercising we will start to enjoy it as a matter of course.

Even thinking about the fact that we will be feeling better through exercise will boost the production of dopamine. If you succeed in focusing on the positive results it will become easier to force yourself to start moving.

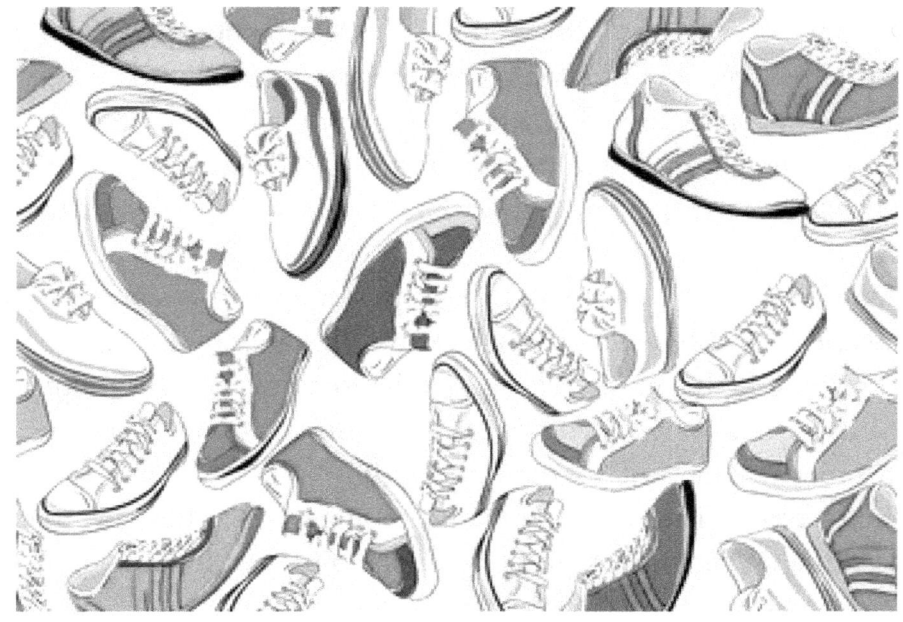

(© richcat – Fotolia.com)

After a while, people fall back into old, unhealthy habits and find it hard to put on their sports shoes. Some tricks may help to change behaviour permanently.

Weakness

Many people have the good intentions and even transform them into healthy behaviour for a time. But after a while they fall back into their old, unhealthy habits. It is very hard to break this pattern.

Here are some key steps in changing behaviour.
- When you start exercising don't overdo it.

- Playing music creates a stimulating environment and enhances the motivation to exercise.

- Lay out smart, specific goals that are attainable.

- Give yourself a reward for reaching one of your goals. This will motivate you to reach for the next goal.

- Don't be too harsh on yourself, but know your weaknesses and try to stay ahead of them. If you don't want to go to the gym today because you are dead tired, give yourself a break and be lazy for once. But make sure tomorrow you will go to the gym! If you don't you probably won't go the day after tomorrow or the following day.

- Believe in your capability to maintain your new, healthy behaviour.

People are prone to act against their better judgment. This weakness of the will is still an unsolved problem. Consciously and unconsciously, at every moment we choose between good things now and better things later. Most people choose a small reward at once instead of a large reward afterwards.
The brain must possess a mechanism to weigh opportunities and risks of different choices, estimate our longevity and tune emotions accordingly. With different kinds of motives fighting within us, the spirit is willing, but the flesh is weak.
According to American psychologist Steven Pinker, some urge to indulge now must have been built into our emotions.

CONCLUSION

The golden recipe

From the moment we are born, the single certainty we have in life is that we will die, sooner or later. For most people, the moment of death will come at advanced age. Of course, everybody would prefer to live a long and healthy life and at the end, a very short period of decline that leads to a rapid death.

Nobody likes getting older. To age gracefully is all about letting nature take its course. We have to start by simply accepting the fact that we will age and eventually will die. In some societies where people still live in a more natural way, these facts are incorporated in everyday life. Western societies have increasingly succeeded in turning ageing and dying into taboos which shouldn't be talked about and should be kept hidden. Thanks to for instance cosmetic surgery the myth of eternal youth has taken on a preposterous form and is accompanied by the illusion of eternal life.

Only young and healthy people seem to matter nowadays in western societies. We don't grant our seniors the special status and privileges they have in other parts of the world. Elsewhere, elderly are being honoured for their wisdom. In our societies, the image of senior citizens only deteriorates. They are too slow and need walkers and mobility scooters to move about. They are suffering many diseases and generate huge costs for society. The fact that governments and media only talk about the problems and costs of the sharp increase in the ageing population isn't contributing to a more positive image of senior citizens either. Consequently, the general public has come to judge the elderly as problematic.

In times gone by, grandparents were old people in the true sense of the word. They sat on their chairs, gave their grandchildren a little pat on the head and a candy and that was it. They died in their sixties or seventies. When they were very tough they possibly reached their eighties.

Modern-day grandparents often are quite different. They don't look like the stereotyped old people in rocking chairs anymore. They dress nicely, feel young-at-heart, take their grandchildren to the amusement park, know what is going on in the world, and can be contacted via their mobile phones and their Facebook pages. And they can easily reach their eighties and nineties. Many of them even go past one hundred.

People's fear of ageing is often greater than necessary. Ageing isn't synonymous with general decline. This only happens when something is wrong, when some kind of pathological process is going on. Through a healthy lifestyle it is possible to avoid or delay the onset of age-related diseases.

How you think about your age may actually affect how you age. For ten years, researchers in the US followed about five hundred people aged 55 and older. It turned out subjective age has a stronger effect on cognitive abilities than chronological age. Elderly people who felt old experienced more decline. The ones who kept a sense of being younger, showed greater confidence about their cognitive abilities and maintained these. This is good news, as research in Germany showed people over 70 years of age on average tend to feel about thirteen years younger than their chronological age.

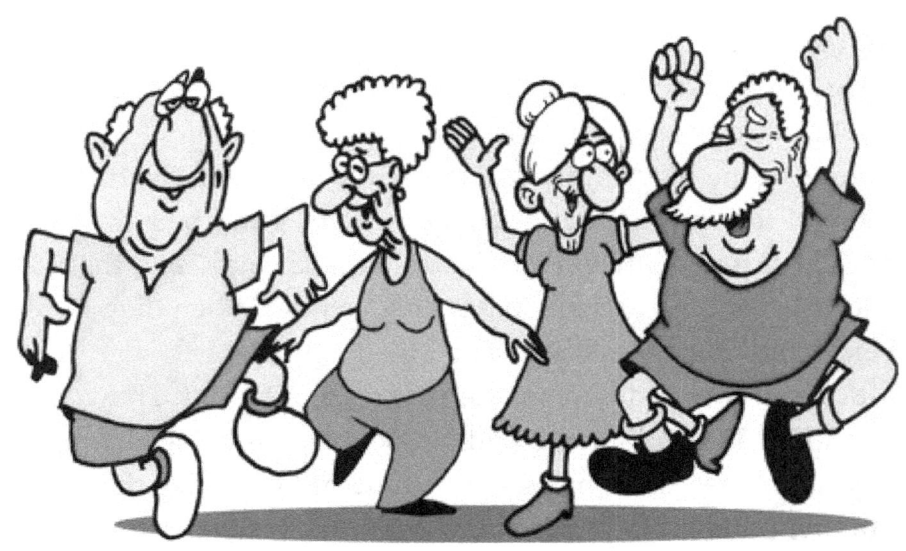

(© Bello - Fotolia.com)

Feel young and be younger.

Choices

It seems we already have a lot of possibilities to be ageing healthy and happily. Everyone can make choices about how to age. Instead of complaining about what you have lost you should focus on what you still can do, find ways to perform well, and compensate for any age-related loss. Doing things one finds meaningful and maintaining control over one's life are very important factors in ageing well.

Yet all too often the advice falls on deaf ears. We don't go for the choices that would be best for our health. One of the reasons for this is that the longer we live the more we get stuck in routine. Older people become less flexible. Their lives tend to become full of habits. They stick to a daily grind and feel comfortable this way. Familiar types of stimulation turn out to be more pleasurable.

For many years, older adults have been socialising with the same friends and acquaintances. They are inclined to associate with like-minded individuals as information that does not match their beliefs and perception of the world can be felt as distressing and difficult to handle.

The organisation of the brain contributes to the ease of taking the beaten tracks, so you have to counteract this inflexibility with conscious effort. You have to undertake new activities and be open to new contacts.

Besides, a lack of motivation may keep you from maintaining or improving your health situation. It is important to find that motivation within yourself. The essence is to change your pattern of movement, your pattern of eating or your pattern of behaviour because you want to do so, not because other people impose such a change on you. If you are not convinced of your personal advantage you won't be able to sustain the change.

There is reason in the saying "the road to hell is paved with good intentions". To be able to transform good intentions into lasting good behaviour self-control is indispensable. Some simple steps may improve your ability to control yourself. It is very important to notice the results of your efforts. You also have to learn to recognise and control destructive behaviour, like eating sweets when you feel down or falling down on the couch and staying there when you get home from work. Find things that might help you overcome such weak moments, such as watching a funny movie to cheer yourself up or treating yourself to a nice meal after you have done your exercise.

Healthy behaviour appears to be contagious. Researchers found that social norms are the most powerful, but least visible form of social control over human behaviour. When observing others engaging in physical activity or eating behaviours, they seem socially desirable. That's why you increase your chances of success when you adapt your lifestyle together with one or more other persons. In addition, a bit of well-meant pressure from your companions may just be sufficient to make you change your mind and put on your sports shoes anyway.

Thoughts

Especially in undertaking healthy behaviours, thinking you can and will succeed is critical for ultimate success. To make the change to your lifestyle permanent, it is essential you firmly believe in your ability to bring the change about. You should also be convinced the effort will bear fruit. As it happens, our thoughts can not only exert a positive influence on our brain, but also a negative one. When you think you can't do something this thought often proves to be correct, first and foremost because you won't even try.

In psychology, this is called a self-fulfilling prophecy. People come to behave in ways that confirm their own or other's expectations. If you no longer believe you can do something, then you may not even try. Reduced self-confidence about sexual performance will result in an actual reduction in sexual activity. Fatigue because of a lower physical efficacy will lead to the curtailing of physical activities.

General prevalent views can also bring about self-fulfilling prophecies. People's beliefs and expectations about memory indeed turn out to play a role in their actual memory. While getting older, people begin to worry about every memory lapse they have. Forgetting something from time to time occurs to everyone, young and old. Not only will you block your memory with anxiety about the state of your memory and make yourself forget, but these thoughts will also turn into a self-fulfilling prophecy. Every little thing you can't remember momentarily is immediately attributed to getting older and thus confirms the prejudice.

Research has demonstrated negative stereotypes about ageing and memory loss, influence performance negatively. Elderly people with more positive views of ageing perform significantly better on memory tests.

Medicines

Expectations also matter a lot in the use of medicines. People often aren't too pleased with their doctor if they visit him because of certain symptoms and he doesn't prescribe some medicines. Expectations can be so strong that fake medicines may remove the symptoms. This is called the placebo effect. A placebo is a neutral substance given in the place of an active medicine. It looks like a medicine, but does not contain active ingredients. Placebos are used in research, to compare the effects of real medicines, and by physicians who want to treat a complaint by suggestion. Several studies have shown a placebo can actually have the same results as a medicine. Hence the placebo effect: the belief in recovery can by itself bring about the recovery.

Research has shown placebos are just as effective as real medicines for instance in treating pain and depression. Generally, patients do not know they are receiving a placebo instead of an active medicine. In a study, patients with irritable bowel syndrome were told beforehand they were going to receive a placebo. Even in this situation without deception, the participants in the placebo group showed a significantly higher improvement than the ones in the group that received no treatment. This shows the importance of expectation. If we expect our health to improve, it often does. The placebo effect is an excellent example of the healing power of the brain.

It would be of great importance to conduct further research into placebos as they may limit the necessity for medicines. Especially the elderly use many different drugs for various ailments. Side effects often bring about the need for more medicines. It would be healthy if they could take a harmless placebo as an alternative for some disorders. This wouldn't be an option for patients with dementia though. As they generally have reduced expectations about medication due to their mental situation, the effects of treatment with a placebo will also be reduced.

The custom of prescribing medicines is very widespread. In the US, of the people between 45 and 64 years old more than 65 percent have been using prescription drugs in the last thirty days. In people over 65 this rises to almost 90 percent. Almost 35 percent of people between 45 and 64 have been using three or more prescription drugs and in people over 65 this was more than 65 percent. And even when looking at five or more prescription drugs percentages are still high: almost 17 and almost 40 respectively.

Not only is the doctor rather quick in prescribing medicines, but we also prefer to take the easy way ourselves when it comes to our health by going for the pills, the injections, the operations, the miracle diet, and so on. Very often this easy way is far from the best way. Just one tiny example: recently, it has been discovered a medicine to quit smoking increases the risk of a heart attack or a stroke. In this case, the remedy is worse than the problem.

Far too easily, elderly people are persuaded to take – often not yet absolutely necessary - medication in situations where a bit of extra attention would work just as well. Medical aids, like walkers and mobility scooters that have become available in recent times – in several countries fully subsidised - are handed out like hot cakes. Of course they are great tools when you can't walk without support anymore. But in many cases, it would be far healthier urging the older adults to make an effort to try to keep on walking a bit more or try to manage only with a walking stick. Rather than having their legs degenerate rapidly due to immobility, they would be able to enjoy their use for a longer period still. On top of that they would help their brains stay healthy thanks to the physical activity. An extremely important factor in ageing well is maintaining a degree of independence and control over one's life. A strong sense of personal freedom is critical to surviving in good health to a ripe age.

It is high time we stop running to the doctor or going to the pharmacy to buy miracle cures in the expectation they will solve our problems. First and foremost, we should take responsibility for our own life and our own health. After all, we know ourselves best, don't we? In many instances, we actually know what the trouble is. Shouldn't we eat some more fruits and vegetables? Shouldn't we try to relax a bit more? And above all, shouldn't we start to exercise far more?

Emotions
Thoughts, emotions, and attitudes play a critical role in how you age. Quite a few elderly are worrying a lot and are down-

hearted regularly. This influences the ageing process negatively. Strong links exist between mood and health. Improving mood lowers pain, curbs anxiety, and improves the quality of life. A good mood boosts immune system functioning and may influence longevity. Flexibility and humour are attitudes associated with healthy ageing.

It is common knowledge that to laugh is very good for you. Laughter brings about profound changes in many parts of the body. It relaxes muscles, increases blood flow to the peripheries, and stimulates the production of neurotransmitters like dopamine. Children laugh at least 400 times a day; grown-ups on average don't do it more than 25 times a day.

But telling someone they have to laugh more is easier said than done. Those who want to abandon themselves to the positive effects of laughter can go to laughter therapy sessions. During these sessions, participants at first produce a kind of forced chuckle, but soon change to a real laughter and end up roaring with laughter, because laughing is so contagious. These bursts of laughter can last up to 20 minutes. At the end of the session, everybody feels great. Laughter yoga originated in India in 1995. Now, more than 8,000 laughter clubs exist in 65 countries.

Motor systems in the brain are involved in emotions as well. There's an extraordinary exchange between the two. Emotions stimulate physical expressions. When you're happy, facial muscles pull your mouth into a smile. But the process also functions the other way around. Physical expressions evoke the matching emotions. When you stretch your facial muscles to form a smile you will feel happier. Thus the movement of facial muscles can improve your mood.

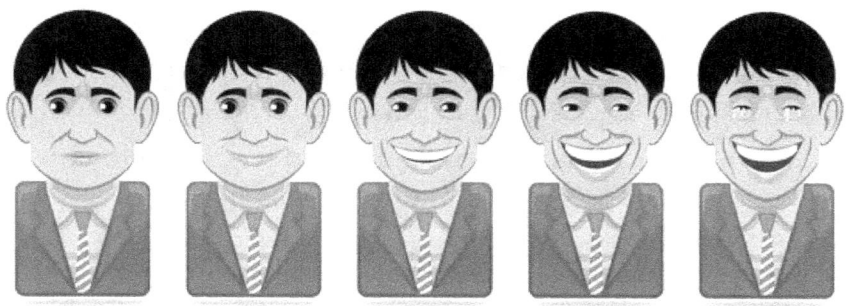

Facial muscles influence our mood. Activating the facial muscles for smiling will actually make you feel more cheerful.

German scientists have proven this two-way traffic through an interesting experiment. About eighty university students participated in the experiment. They were divided into two groups. All of the participants were given a pen. One group was instructed to hold the pen with their lips. This activates the facial muscles you will also use when frowning. The second group was instructed to hold the pen with their teeth. This activates the muscles used for smiling.

Then, the participants were shown a series of cartoons. The students who had the pen between their teeth and thus were simulating a smile, thought the cartoons considerably funnier than the students with the pen between their lips, simulating a frown.

Since it has become clear our facial muscles influence our mood, scientists are interested in the consequences of using the currently very popular Botox injections to counteract wrinkles. Botox causes a temporal paralysis of the facial muscles used in frowning. The first results of research into these consequences indicate that after injecting Botox a dampening of activity occurs in the brain parts involved in processing emotions. Further studies have to be done to find out whether Botox hampers the ability to react emotionally. Anger and hostility cause exactly the opposite effects of cheerfulness and laughing. They even increase the risk of heart attacks and strokes.

To regulate mood, suppression and rumination are counterproductive. They make a negative mood worse. More effective is looking for distraction to make the bad mood fade away. Humour is the most powerful of self-control processes.

Happiness

If you are inclined to think negatively about life, you can actively work towards a more positive attitude. Set out to see the glass as half-full instead of as half-empty. Express your feelings so you can deal with them. Open up your heart to someone. Don't take little annoyances too seriously. Try to see the joke of something, even in difficult circumstances. Start with putting a smile on your face a bit more often.

The good news is that life satisfaction and happiness in general do not decline with age.

On the contrary, surveys show older adults generally are happier than younger adults. They have more health problems, but fewer problems overall.

Elderly people feel less pressured to achieve and succeed and have more time for leisurely pursuits. People have fewer negative emotions and more positive ones compared to when they were younger. Maturity brings more emotional stability. This doesn't mean ageing will turn someone who has been a grumpy person all of his life into a happy one. But most people will gradually feel better as they grow older

Humans have a considerable capacity for adaptation. Even in the most adverse circumstances, many people are able to adapt and get something positive out of the negative. Thanks to their lifelong experience, the elderly are particularly good at this.

An important factor in happiness is sexuality. Orgasms are accompanied by a surge in hormones that cause the brain to create feelings of happiness.

Due to ageing, changes in sexual performance occur. These changes are stronger in males, who may have problems getting or keeping erections and who may experience less frequent orgasms.

Sexual activity, a good quality sex life, and interest in sex are positively associated with health. Crucial factors for an extended sex life are regularity and opportunity. Societies often still treat sex between elderly as a taboo. But sexual activity can continue throughout one's life, so long as the belief that old people are or should be asexual doesn't interfere. Sex reconfirms feelings shared between people regardless of age.

Clear

Now that we know a little bit about what is going on in our brain, the message is clear: if we want to keep our cognitive abilities functioning well into old age, we have to start and keep on moving! Movement is inseparably tied to cognition. Cognitive functions have evolved from movement and still depend on it. Physical activity is vital to all brain functions, including learning and memory. A lot of brain function is in essence movement. It's no coincidence interesting thoughts pop up in your head when taking a walk or working out on some exercise machine.

That is why physical exercise is the most important activity for body and brain fitness. It enhances cerebral blood flow, which tends to diminish while ageing and it improves glucose utilisation. These two factors alone can do a lot of good for the ageing brain. But also on the cellular level, physical exercise brings about many positive changes, among which an increase in the availability of neurotransmitters.

The annoying thing of the matter is that moving is just the one activity we have been engaging in less and less. So we have to find other ways to give our brain the movement it needs. We have to free up time to consciously start moving. For the generalised improvement in brain function and capacity to come about, it has to be rigorous, aerobic exercise for at least half an hour, five times a week. And it is a job that never ends, because some time after quitting the exercise, the benefits will disappear as well. Make it a life-long commitment!

Star

The right amount of exercise is extremely beneficial to the small brain structure called hippocampus. The hippocampus is a star player in our efforts to keep our brain healthy as long as possible. It is one of the known parts in the adult brain where new neurogenesis - the birth of new neurones - continues to take place and it plays a crucial role in learning and memory. In a brain suffering from dementia, the hippocampus is one of the first parts to deteriorate and it is also the part that is hit hardest. A healthy, robust hippocampus helps to stave off dementia.

To give the hippocampus a helping hand in its many duties, the first thing to do is try to avoid stress at all cost and learn to cope rapidly with the stress you do experience to minimise damage. Chronic stress inhibits the birth of new neurones, reduces the volume of the hippocampus, and leads to impaired memory.

So it is a matter of the utmost importance to take good care of the hippocampus, in the first place, by exercising sufficiently, and in the second place, by de-stressing. Try to relax by means of breathing techniques, yoga, reading a good book, or whatever other way suits you most.

To aid the memory function of the hippocampus you may take some practical steps.

- Give what you want to store in memory all your attention. Take away as many distractions as possible.

- Organise a positive atmosphere while studying what you want to remember. Emotions exert an important influence on your memory.

- Make sure you sleep well. While sleeping, connections made during the day are repeated. This helps to store memories.

Consistent with the favourable influence of movement on the hippocampus, researchers concluded taking a walk will reinforce memory. It is best to go for a walk out in the country side where you'll encounter fewer distractions so you can concentrate better.

Apart from physical exercise, mental exercise is very useful as well to activate the hippocampus. Learning new things and going through enriched experiences promote the making of contacts between neurones.

As mentioned before, I think it is not worth it to spend money on expensive brain training programs. Apart from engaging people in some interesting activities, brain training programs so far do not result in what their makers are promising. They do improve performance on the specific tasks tackled by the programs, but this does not lead to generalised effects. Far more helpful is for instance learning another language.

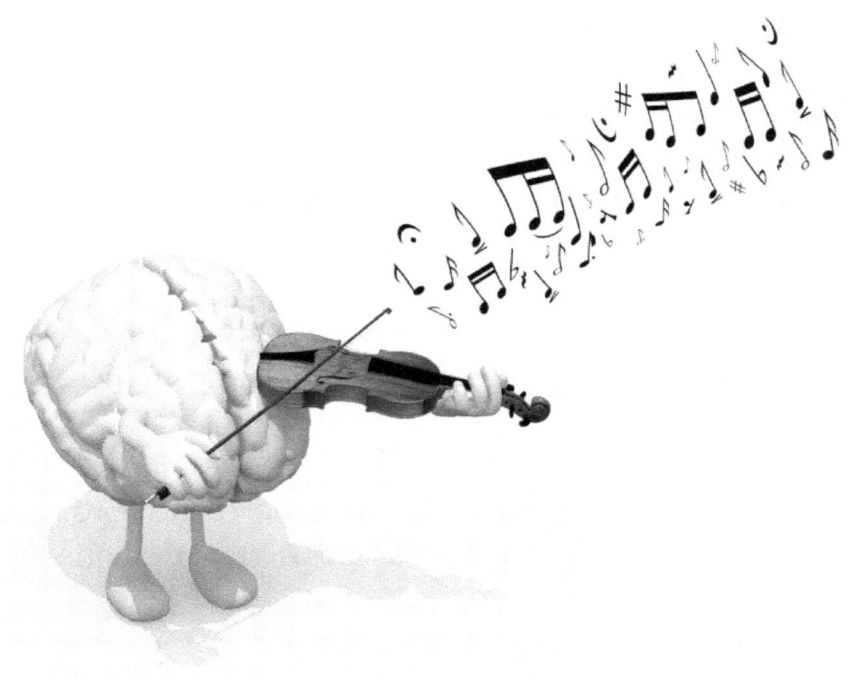

(© fabioberti.it - Fotolia.com)

Playing a musical instrument is the best activity to enhance your brain fitness. It activates large parts of the brain and brings into being many new neural networks.

Music

The golden opportunity to enhance your brain fitness is learning to play a musical instrument. Making music activates large parts of the brain and brings into being many new neural networks.

Your goal shouldn't be to end up on the number one spot of the pop charts, but just to enjoy yourself. Or maybe to even find pleasure with some other players since social contact also benefits the brain.

The proverbial phrase 'you are never too old to learn' is true also for learning to play a musical instrument. It is after all not about how proficient you will become but about the benefits you will gain and about the pleasure making music will provoke.

Dancing is also an excellent brain activity due to the series of movements that need you to think very hard too.

Of course plenty of other activities exist to keep an active mind, like reading an interesting book.

You could solve puzzles for instance, but don't let it be the same old crossword puzzle all the time. Change to a Sudoku or a jigsaw puzzle every now and then.

If you like computer games, agility games are another possibility. In your scores, you will notice an improvement while playing, which means you are training that part of your brain that is activated for playing this particular game.

Another type of game will activate neurones and stimulate new connections in another part of your brain.

Surfing the internet makes good practice for your brain as well, according to an American study among groups of seniors who did or did not use the internet.

Changes

Even in your daily routine you can keep on stimulating your brain. Routine is a good thing. It brings rest and regularity into daily activities and offers grip especially in old age. But too many fixed habits are bad. The brain switches to the automatic pilot and becomes 'lazy'.

On a small scale, you can make changes in your daily activities. Take a look at your dressing routine for example. To put your first sock on your left foot and then the other one on your right foot can also be done the other way around. To do it differently you have to do it consciously. And that is good for the brain!

More difficult and thus more effective is using a different hand than usual. If you always pick up things with your right hand try to do it with your left hand next time. To write with a different hand from the one you are used to, is very hard, but even trying to write with your other hand once in a while can create new connections.

Your fixed routine of fitness exercises or the fixed walk with the dog can also be done in a different sequence. Everybody has this kind of fixed habits that could be done a little different. It is important over time to stay focused on your habits to not let the new sequence become the next routine.

Cultural activities like going to the theatre, the cinema or an exhibition have a positive influence on your well-being and at the same time activate your brain in a useful manner.

Socialising with other people also plays a role in brain training. But you need to be open to other people's stories, ideas, and opinions and not only want to ventilate your own stories. Other people can have a very healthy influence on your habitual, maybe somewhat inflexible perspective. Your neurones regroup to adapt your own ideas and opinions a little.

In short, it is extremely important to keep an open mind for 'new' in all kinds of areas, even though this is hard since most people become more rigid when they get older.

Joy

It is obvious a healthy diet is vital to body and brain fitness. What we eat is fundamental to how we think and feel. The appropriate amounts of all nutrients should come from a variety of fruits, vegetables, nuts, and spices, preferably fresh and as less cooked as possible.

They should be accompanied by an adequate amount of water. We have a tendency to take it a bit too easy when it comes to the appropriate amounts. It is of the utmost importance to eat at least five servings of fruits and vegetables day, preferably more.

As for coffee, three cups is the preferred limit per day, and for alcoholic beverages, two glasses per day for men and one for women. Feel free to drink a glass of red wine daily since it is good for your brain; only don't do that late in the evening as this will work out badly for your REM sleep. And don't forget to go out in the sun regularly to get sufficient vitamin D, a shortage of which increases the risk of stroke and dementia. There's no unambiguous answer yet to the question whether the positive results would be the same by taking supplements containing for instance vitamins, minerals, or antioxidants. That's why it's best to get them from the food you eat, except in special cases when someone suffers a considerable shortage and supplementing might be necessary.

One of the things we don't have to worry about anymore at

an advanced age is those few pounds surplus of body weight we may carry. It turned out by that time such a surplus doesn't make a difference in your health situation. You don't have to bother losing a lot of weight to live longer. In fact, considerable calorie restriction not only is unrealistic, but it also appears to have a negative influence on longevity in older adults.

Besides, it would take away a lot of joy in life, which comes from eating - preferably in good company to reap the benefits of social contacts on brain health - and which contributes to well-being as well.

The same goes true for all activities that have passed in review. In the end, it is you who has to find the best way for you to live a healthy lifestyle. Whether you are satisfied with your life appears to have a crucial effect on the health of your brain at later age.

And now

At the end of this book, you have a bit of an idea what your brain looks like. You have caught a glimpse of how the brain and the genes operate – at least, what we now know of their functioning so far.

You also know your brain, even though it is safely tucked away in your skull, is constantly exposed to influences from outside. Which activities you undertake, what foods you eat, and where you are located, not only shape your brain, but play a role in the functioning of your genes as well.

Even if you would live exactly by the book and thus do the right things, follow the healthy diet, and avoid unhealthy environments, it wouldn't guarantee a healthy brain with all its mental powers right until the moment of your death.

That is possibly because there are other processes going on in the brain which we still don't know. Besides, the influences that affect your brain start very early, namely in the first environment you are living in: your mother's womb.
But it is certain that you will considerably increase your chances of a healthy brain at advanced age by sticking to a healthy lifestyle. And it is never too early or too late to start with that. So start living brain-consciously now!

Armed with the knowledge in this book, you can draw up a plan of action. What are your weaknesses and how will you tackle them?

Those who prefer a more practical approach may go about creating their personal brain-conscious lifestyle in the following manner.
Take a random day of your life. At the end of that day, write down all the things you have done on that ordinary day.

- How many hours did I sleep last night and what was the quality of my sleep? Did I get out of bed well-rested?

- What did I eat during the day?

- Did I stimulate my brain today by doing challenging things, by undertaking something new, by making contacts?

- Did I experience stress today? How much and in which situations?

- Did I get my aerobic exercise today? For how long?

Then take this book. Go to the chapters concerned and find out whether your answers to these questions coincide with the recommendations for a healthy lifestyle.

The next question will then be in how many areas you would need to improve your lifestyle.

Next, make your choice which area you want to take on first and how you will go about adapting your lifestyle to the recommendations for that area.

Write down your goals and preferably add a time frame in which you want to reach every goal. In doing so, try to be realistic since nothing is more demotivating than goals you didn't make.

This way, step by step, you will get to your brain-conscious lifestyle.

BIBLIOGRAPHY

Agata, Kyokazu (2008). Planaria nervous system.
www.scholarpedia.org/article/Planaria_nervous_system
Aimone, James B. & Jessberger, Sebastian & Gage, Fred H. (2007).
Adult neurogenesis. www.scholarpedia.org/article/
Adult_neurogenesis
Attix, Deborah K. & Welsh-Bohmer, Kathleen A. (2006). Geriatric
neuropsychology, assessment and intervention. New York: The
Guilford Press.
Bains, Jaideep S. & Oliet, Stéphane H.R. (2007). Glia: they make
your memories stick. Trends in neurosciences, 30(8), 417-424.
Barnes, L.L. & Mendes de Leon, C.F. & Wilson, R.S. & Blenisa, J.L. &
Evans, D.A. (2004). Social resources and cognitive decline in a
population of older African Americans and whites. Neurology,
December, 2322-2326.
Beaumont, J. Graham and Pamela M. Kenealy and Marcus J.C.
Rogers (2001). The Blackwell Dictionary of Neuropsychology.
Oxford: Blackwell Publishers.
Bjelakovic, Goran & Nikalova, Dimitrinka & Gluud, Lise Lotte &
Simonetti, Rosa G. & Gluud, Christian (2007). Mortality in
randomized trials of antioxidant supplements for primary and
secondary prevention. Jama, 28 February, 842-857.
Blackmore, Susan (2006). Conversations on consciousness: what the
best minds think about the brain, free will, and what it means to be
human. New York: Oxford University Press.
Bloom, Floyd & Flint Beal, M. & Kupfer, David J. (2006). The Dana
guide to brain health: a practical family reference from medical
experts. New York: Dana Press.
Bolte Taylor, Jill (2006). My stroke of insight, a brain scientist's
personal journey. New York: Viking Penguin.
Boyke, Janina & Driemeyer, Joenna & Gaser, Christian e.a. (2008).

Training-induced brain structure changes in the elderly. The Journal of Neuroscience, 9 July, 7031-7035.

Brodal, Per (2010). The central nervous system. New York: Oxford University Press.

Bryson, Bill (2003). A short history of nearly everything. New York: Broadway Books.

Bryson, Bill (2010). Seeing further: the story of science, discover & the genius of the Royal Society. New York: HarperCollins Publishers.

Buchman, Aron S. & Boyle, Patricia A. & Wilson, Robert S. & Fleischman, Debra A. & Leurgans, Sue & Bennett, David A. (2009). Association between late-life social activity and motor decline in older adults. Archives of Internal Medicine, June,1139-1146.

Carey, Joseph (2005). Brain Facts, a primer on the brain and nervous system. Washington: Society for Neuroscience.

Carlson, Michelle C. (2011). Promoting healthy, meaningful aging through social involvement: building an experience corps. Cerebrum, June, http://dana.org/news/cerebrum/

Carpentier, Pamela A. & Palmer, Theo D. (2009). Immune influence on adult neural stem cell regulation and function. Neuron, 15 October, 79-92.

Carter, Rita (2002). Exploring consciousness. Berkeley: University of California Press.

Chopra, Deepak (1993). Ageless body, timeless mind: the quantum alternative to growing old. New York: Harmony Books.

Coon, Dennis (2004). Introduction to psychology: gateways to mind and behavior. Belmont: Thomson Wadsworth.

Cooper, Jack R. & Bloom, Floyd E. & Roth, Robert H. (2003). The biochemical basis of neuropharmacology 8th ed. New York: Oxford University Press.

Coren, Stanley (1997). Sleep Thieves, an eye-opening exploration into the science and mysteries of sleep. New York: Free Press Paperbacks.

Crick, Francis (1994). The astonishing hypothesis: the scientific search for the soul. New York: Touchstone.

Csikszentmihalyi, Mihaly (1990). Flow, the psychology of optimal experience – steps toward enhancing the quality of life. New York: HarperCollins Publishers.

Damasio, Antonio R. (1994). Descartes' error: emotion, reason, and the human brain. New York: HarperCollins Publishers.

Damasio, Antonio R. (1999). The feeling of what happens: body and emotion in the making of consciousness. Orlando: Harcourt.

Damasio, Antonio R. (2003). Looking for Spinoza: joy, sorrow, and the feeling brain. Orlando: Harcourt.

Darwin, Charles (2001). On the origin of species. Cambridge: Harvard University Press.

Descartes, René (1989). Discourse on method and the meditations. New York: Prometheus Books.

Diamond, M.C. and A.B. Scheibel and L.M. Elson (1985). The human brain coloring book. New York: HarperCollins Publishers.

Doidge, Norman (2007). The brain that changes itself. New York: Penguin Books.

Douglas Field R. (2011). The other brain: the scientific and medical breakthroughs that will heal our brains and revolutionize our health. New York: Simon & Schuster.

Edelman, Gerald M. & Tononi, Giulio (2000). A universe of consciousness: how matter becomes imagination. New York: Basic Books.

Eichenbaum, Howard. Memory. www.scholarpedia.org/article/ Memory

Encyclopaedia Britannica (2008). The brain, a guided tour of the brain – mind, memory, and intelligence. London: Constable & Robinson.

Ertel, Karen A. & Glymour, M. Maria & Berkman, Lisa F. (2008). Effects of social integration on preserving memory function in a nationally representative US elderly population. American Journal of Public Health, July, 1215-1220.

Figuero, Mariana G. & Bierman, Andrew & Bullough, John D. & Rea, Mark S. (2009). A personal light-treatment device for improving sleep quality in elderly: dynamics of nocturnal melatonin suppression at two exposure levels. Chronobiology International, January.

Gazzaniga, Michael S. (1998). The mind's past. Berkeley: University of California Press.

Gazzaniga, Michael S. & Heatherton, Todd F. (2003). Psychological science: mind, brain, and behavior. New York: W.W. Norton & Company.

Gazzaniga, Michael S. (2008). Human: the science behind what makes us unique. New York: HarperCollins Publishers.

Gazzaniga, Michael S. & Ivry, Richard B. & Mangun, George R. (2009). Cognitive Neuroscience, the biology of the mind 3rd ed. New York: W.W. Norton & Company.

Gazzaniga, Michael S. (2012). Who's in charge? Free will and the science of the brain. New York: Ecoo.

Goldberg, Elkhonon (2001). The executive brain: frontal lobes and the civilized mind. New York: Oxford University Press.

Goldberg, Elkhonon (2005). The wisdom paradox: how your mind can grow stronger as your brain grows older. New York: Gotham Books.

Gould, Stephen Jay (2002). The structure of evolutionary theory. Cambridge: Harvard University Press.

Gregory, Richard L. (2004). The Oxford companion to the mind. Oxford: Oxford University Press.

Havas, David A. & Glenberg, Arthur M. & Gutowski, Karol A. & Lucarelli, Mark J. & Davidson, Richard J. (2010). Cosmetic use of botulinum toxin-A affects processing of emotional language. Psychological Science, July, 895-900.

Hazen, Robert M. & Trefil, James (1991). Science matters, achieving scientific literacy. New York: Anchor Books.

Hennenlotter, Andreas & Dresel, Christian & Castrop, Florian & Ceballos-Baumann, Andres O. & Wohlschlager, Afra M. & Haslinger, Bernhard (2009). The link between facial feedback and neural activity within central circuitries of emotion - new insights from botulinum toxin-induced denervation of frown muscles. Cerebral Cortex, March, 537-542.

Hoang, MinhTu T. & DeFina, Laura F. & Willis, Benjamin L. & Leonard, David S. & Weiner, Myron F. & Sherwood Brown, E. (2011). Association between low serum 25-hydroxyvitamin D and depression in a large sample of healthy adults: the Cooper Center longitudinal study. Mayo Clinic Proceedings, November, 1050-1055.

Howard, Pierce (2001). The owner's manual for the brain. Atlanta: Bard Press.

James, B.D. & Wilson, R.S. & Barnes, L.L. & Bennett, D.A. (2011). Late-life social activity and cognitive decline in old age. Journal of the International Neuropsychological Society, November, 998-1005.

Joseph, James & Cole, Greg & Head, Elizabeth e.a. (2009). Nutrition, brain aging, and neurodegeneration. The Journal of Neuroscience, 14 October, 12795-12801.

Kandel, Eric R. & Schwartz, James H. & Jessell, Thomas M. (2000). Principles of Neural Science 4th ed. New York: McGraw-Hill.

Kokovay, Ersebet & Shen, Qin & Temple, Sally (2008). The incredible elastic brain: how neural stem cells expand our minds. Neuron, 6 November, 420-429.

Koob, Andrew (2009). The root of thought: unlocking glia, the brain cell that will help us sharpen our wits, heal injury, and treat brain disease. Upper Saddle River: FT Press.

Kramer, Arthur F. & Erickson, Kirk I. & Colcombe, Stanley J. (2006). Exercise, cognition, and the aging brain. Journal of Applied Physiology, June, 1237-1242.

Laming, Peter R. & Sykova, Eva & Reichenbach, Andres e.a. (2010). Glial cells: their role in behaviour. Cambridge: Cambridge University Press.

LeDoux, Joseph E (2002). Synaptic Self: how our brains become who we are. New York: Viking Penguin.

Lezak, Muriel D. & Howieson, Diane B. & Loring, David W. (2004). Neuropsychological assessment 4th ed. New York: Oxford University Press.

Loring, David W. (1999). INS dictionary of neuropsychology. New York: Oxford University Press.

Lucas, Michael & Mekary, Rania & Pan, An & Mirzael, Fariba & O'Reilly, Ellis J. & Willett, Walter C. & Koenen, Karestan & Okereke, Olivia I. & Ascherlo, Alberto (2011). Relation between clinical depression risk and physical activity and time spent watching television in older women: a 10-year prospective follow-up study. American Journal of Epidemiology, October, 1017-1027.

Lucin, Kurt M. & Wyss-Coray, Tony (2009). Immune activation in brain aging and neurodegeneration; too much or too little? Neuron, 15 October, 110-122.

Mattson, Mark P. (2008). Glutamate and neurotrophic factors in neuronal plasticity and disease. Annals of the New York Academy of Sciences, November, 97-112.

Myers, D. (2007). Psychology of happiness. www.scholarpedia.org/article/Psychology_of_happiness

Nofzinger, Eric & Buysse, Daniel (2011). Cooling the brain during sleep may be an easy, natural and effective treatment for insomnia. American Academy of Sleep Medicine, June, news release.

Noordam, Raymond & Gunn, David A, & Tomlin, Cyrena C, & Maier, Andrea B. & Mooiaart, Simon P. & Slagboom, P. Eline & Westendorp, Rudi G.J. & de Craen, Anton J.M. & van Heemst, Diana (2013). High serum glucose levels are associated with a higher perceived age. Age, February, 189-195.

Pasley, Brian N. & Freeman, Ralph D. (2008). Neurovascular coupling. www.scholarpedia.org/article/Neurovascular_coupling

Pinker, Steven (1997). How the mind works. New York: W.W. Norton & Company.

Ramachandran, Vilayanur S. (2004). A brief tour of human consciousness. New York: Pi Press.

Ratey, John J. (2002). A user's guide to the brain: perception, attention, and the four theaters of the brain. New York: Vintage Books.

Ratey, John J. & Hagerman, Eric (2008). Spark: the revolutionary new science of exercise and the brain. New York: Little, Brown and Company.

Redgrave, Peter (2007). Basal Ganglia. www.scholarpedia.org/article/Basal_ganglia

Ridley, Matt (2000). Genome, the autobiography of a species in 23 chapters. New York: HarperCollins Publishers Inc.

Ridley, Matt (2004). The agile gene: how nature turns on nurture. New York: Harper Perennial.

Ridley, Matt (2010). The rational optimist: how prosperity evolves. New York: HarperCollins Publishers.

Rosenkranz, Karin & Williamon, Aaron & Rothwell, John C. (2007). Motorcortical excitability and synaptic plasticity is enhanced in professional musicians. The Journal of Neuroscience, 9 May, 5200-5206.

Sacks, Oliver (1998). The man who mistook his wife for a hat and other clinical tales. New York: Touchstone.

Santrock, John W.(2006). Life-span development 10th ed. New York: McGraw-Hill.

Schultz, Duane P. and Sydney Ellen Schultz (2005). Theories of personalities 8th ed. Belmont: Thomson Wadsworth.

Schultz, Wolfram (2007). Reward. www.scholarpedia.org/article/Reward

Singh-Manoux, Archana & Kivimaki, Mika & Glymour M. Maria & Elbaz, Alexis & Berr, Claudine & Ebmeier, Klaus P. & Ferrie, Jane E. & Dugravot, Aline (2012). Timing of onset of cognitive decline: results from Whitehall II prospective cohort study. British Medical Journal, January, 344-352.

Smith Churchland, Patricia (2002). Brain-Wise: studies in neurophilosophy. Cambridge: A Bradford Book.

Sontheimer, Harald W. Glial influence on synaptic transmission. Center for Glial Biology in Medicine, University of Alabama, http://glia-uab.infomedia.com/content.asp?id=113345

Spinoza, Benedict de (1996). Ethics. London: Penguin Books.

Squire, Larry R. & Kandel, Eric R. (2009). Memory: from mind to molecules. Greenwood Village: Roberts and Company Publishers.

Strack, Fritz & Martin, Leonard L. & Stepper, Sabine (1988). Inhibiting and facilitating conditions of the human smile: a nonobtrusive test of the facial feedback hypothesis. Journal of Personality and Social Psychology, May, 768-777.

The Dana Alliance for Brain Initiatives (2008). Your brain at work: making the science of cognitive fitness work for you. New York.

The Dana Alliance for Brain Initiatives (2010). Staying sharp, current advances in brain research: successful aging and your brain. New York.

Tononi, Giulio (2012). Phi: a voyage from the brain to the soul. New York: Pantheon.

University of Minnesota. The nun study. www.healthstudies.umn.edu/nunstudy/

Varkey, Emma & Cider, Ada & Carlsson, Jane & Linde, Mattias (2011). Exercise as migraine prophylaxis: a randomized study using relaxation and topiramate as controls. Cephalgia, October, 1428-1438.

Verkhratsky, Alexei & Butt, Arthur (2007). Glial neurobiology, a textbook. Chichester: John Wiley & Sons Ltd.

Villeda, Saul & Wyss-Coray, Tony (2008). Microglia: a wrench in the running wheel? Neuron, 28 August, 527-529.

Watson, James D. (2001). Genes, girls, and Gamow – after the double helix. New York: Vintage Books.

Watson, James D. (2001). The double helix, a personal account of the discovery of the structure of DNA. New York: Touchstone.

Weil, Andrew (2005). Healthy aging. New York: Alfred A. Knopf.

Weil, Andrew (2001). Eating well for optimum health; the essential guide to bringing health and pleasure back to eating. New York: Quill.

Ybarra, Oscar & Winkielman, Piotr & Yeh, Irene & Burnstein, Eugene & Kavanagh, Liam (2011). Friends (and sometimes enemies) with cognitive benefits: what types of social interactions boost executive functioning? Socials Psychology & Personality Science, May, 253-261.

Zillmer, Eric A. & Spiers, Mary V. & Culbertson, William C. (2008). Principles of neuropsychology 2nd ed. Belmont: Thomson.

Alzheimer Research Forum, www.alzforum.org

The brain from top to bottom. http://thebrain.mcgill.ca

The Dana Foundation. www.dana.org

The Journal of Neuroscience. www.jneurosci.org

Wikipedia. www.wikipedia.org